Dental
Materials
A POCKET GUIDE

Dental
Materials
A POCKET GUIDE

KIMBERLY G. BASTIN, CDA, EFDA, RDH, MS
Dental Hygiene Program Director
Sanford-Brown Institute
Jacksonville, Florida

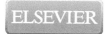

ELSEVIER
SAUNDERS

3251 Riverport Lane
St. Louis, Missouri 63043

DENTAL MATERIALS: A POCKET GUIDE   ISBN: 978-1-4557-4684-2

Notices

Knowledge and best practice in this field are constantly changing. As new research and experience broaden our understanding, changes in research methods, professional practices, or medical treatment may become necessary.

Practitioners and researchers must always rely on their own experience and knowledge in evaluating and using any information, methods, compounds, or experiments described herein. In using such information or methods they should be mindful of their own safety and the safety of others, including parties for whom they have a professional responsibility.

With respect to any drug or pharmaceutical products identified, readers are advised to check the most current information provided (i) on procedures featured or (ii) by the manufacturer of each product to be administered, to verify the recommended dose or formula, the method and duration of administration, and contraindications. It is the responsibility of practitioners, relying on their own experience and knowledge of their patients, to make diagnoses, to determine dosages and the best treatment for each individual patient, and to take all appropriate safety precautions.

To the fullest extent of the law, neither the Publisher nor the authors, contributors, or editors, assume any liability for any injury and/or damage to persons or property as a matter of products liability, negligence or otherwise, or from any use or operation of any methods, products, instructions, or ideas contained in the material herein.

ISBN: 978-1-4557-4684-2

Vice President and Publisher: Linda Duncan
Content Strategist: Kristin Wilhelm
Senior Content Development Specialist: Courtney Sprehe
Publishing Services Manager: Julie Eddy
Project Manager: Jan Waters
Design Direction: Ashley Miner

Printed in the United States of America

Last digit is the print number: 9 8 7 6 5 4 3 2

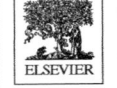

Contents

Message to the Student

This is a dental materials pocket guide. The intention of this guide is to be a simplified version of your dental materials textbooks. The guide will not furnish all of the detail your textbooks do, nor will it provide the detailed information that can be found in manufacturer's instructions, which accompany dental materials. The guide will hopefully refresh your memory of the sequence of steps required to manipulate material when it has been awhile since you have manipulated a specific material. As you begin or continue on your journey in dentistry, you will find there are times you use a specific material on a continual basis, while there are other times you seldom use a material.

As an instructor, I have experienced those times in which students use a material frequently while enrolled in a dental materials course; but do not revisit the manipulation of a material until after summer break. The 3 months the student was off during summer was just long enough for him or her to forget which step comes first when placing a sealant. You may find yourself asking, "do I etch first or clean the tooth with pumice?" Or maybe it has been awhile since you took an alginate impression. You might find yourself asking, "what type of wax were we suppose to use around the edge of an impression tray to make it more comfortable for our patient?"

This guide will not provide all of the answers to the many questions that may arise while manipulating materials. Hopefully, it will jog your memory as to which step comes first and give you some helpful hints for each material. In addition, it is important to remember the directions for the manipulation of materials in this guide are general guidelines. Some manufacturers change sequences for the use of materials to make them brand-specific. A good clinician will always review the manufacturer's instructions before manipulating a material and he or she will always mix the material at least once before using it on a patient.

FOUNDATIONAL CONCEPTS

Manipulation of Dental Materials

The *Dental Materials Pocket Guide* gives you a basic outline of how to handle different dental materials. Manufacturers of dental materials change sequencing of steps on occasion to make a material specific to their company. It is essential to always read the manufacturer's instructions prior to using a material to ensure the proper steps, mixing times, and setting times are followed.

Storage of Dental Materials

The storage of dental materials is very important. Dental materials should always remain in the containers in which they were supplied to the office, unless they are supplied in bulk form. When bulk materials must be transferred to a new container, the new container is considered a secondary container that must be labeled appropriately, and the container in which the material is placed must maintain the integrity of the material. This is important because external factors, such as temperature and humidity, can change the setting reaction of certain dental materials. Some dental materials require refrigeration and should never be stored in the same refrigerator as food. The dental material can leach out of the storage containers and contaminate food if stored in the same refrigerator.

Safety while Using Dental Materials

Safety is an integral part of manipulating dental materials in the dental office or laboratory setting. Universal precautions should be used when manipulating materials, and best practices suggest wearing personal protective equipment inclusive of mask, glasses, lab jacket or overgown, and gloves any time dental materials are going to be manipulated.

Hazards Associated with Dental Materials

Due to the chemical make-up of many dental materials, there are hazards associated with the manipulation of all dental materials. Some of the hazards associated with the use of dental materials are more severe, depending on the composition of the material. It is essential to read the Material Safety Data Sheets (MSDS) that are supplied with the material when it is purchased. The MSDS will provide a description of the physical and chemical properties of the material, any health hazards, routes of exposure, precautions for safe handling and use, first aid and emergency procedures, and spill containment measures. When working with dental materials, it is imperative that a clinician know how to handle an emergency situation and not exacerbate a situation by adding another material that can cause a chemical reaction. The *Dental Materials Pocket Guide* does not indicate the hazards associated with each material, as they can vary depending on the chemical make-up of a material established by the manufacturer.

Infection Control

Infection control measures should be followed in every aspect of providing treatment to patients. It is important to follow the recommended infection control measures established by manufacturers to maintain the integrity of equipment and materials being used within the dental practice. Disposable items should be disposed of after use, and non-disposable items should either be disinfected or sterilized according to the manufacturer's instructions. Critical items that are used to penetrate soft tissue or bone have the greatest risk of transmitting infection and must be sterilized by heat. Semicritical items come in contact with mucous membranes or nonintact skin have a lower risk of transmitting infection, but most are heat-tolerant and should be heat-sterilized when possible.

State Dental Practice Act

Each state has a Dental Practice Act that outlines the rules and regulations governing the practice of dentistry. It is essential for all dental professionals to be versed in the law governing their practice. Some states allow dental assistants and dental hygienists to place restorative materials while other states do not. It is considered malpractice for a dental assistant or dental hygienist to practice according to word-of-mouth without verifying the validity of information provided to them.

Acknowledgments

I would like to acknowledge the following individuals for their assistance with the pocket guide.

*Dr. Wes Booker and Katherine Hite, CDA at Dental Designs of Owensboro, Kentucky. Their willingness to take time out of their busy schedules to provide photos for multiple materials was greatly appreciated.

*Dr. Joslyn Vann, a colleague and friend who allowed me to bounce ideas off of her and provided honest feedback and support.

*To my husband, who became the photographer of most of the materials and always supported me through the process of putting the guide together.

*To the team at Elsevier, especially Kristin Wilhelm and Courtney Sprehe. Your guidance and support is appreciated.

Reference Materials

Bird D, Robinson DS: *Modern Dental Assisting*, ed 11, St. Louis, 2015, Saunders

Boyd LRB: *Dental Instruments: A Pocket Guide*, ed 5, St. Louis, 2015, Saunders

Freedman G: *Contemporary Esthetic Dentistry*, ed 1, St. Louis, 2012, Mosby

Galdwin M, Bagby M: *Clinical Aspects of Dental Materials: Theory, Practice, and Cases*, ed 3, Philadelphia, 2009, Lippincott Williams & Wilkins

Hatrick CD, Eakle WS, Bird WF: *Dental Materials: Clinical Applications for Dental Assistants and Dental Hygienists*, ed 3, St. Louis, 2011, Saunders

Powers JM, Wataha JC: *Dental Materials: Properties and Manipulation*, ed 10, St. Louis, 2013, Mosby

Equipment Commonly Used to Manipulate Materials

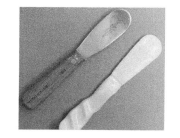

■ **MATERIAL** Flexible Rubber Bowl

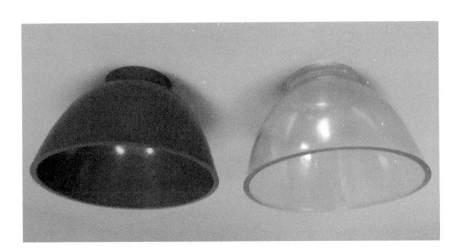

• To mix two materials together, such as a powder and liquid
• To mix impression materials and gypsum products together

Special Notes/Helpful Hints • Disinfect bowls according to manufacturer's instructions. Some disinfectants may break down the composition of the material used to fabricate the bowl. • Bowls should always be disinfected before and after use with a patient.

MATERIAL

Flexible Alginate Spatula

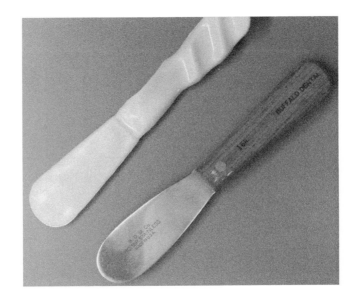

Uses ▶ • To mix two materials together, such as a powder and liquid
• To mix impression materials and gypsum products together

◀▮▶ Special Notes/Helpful Hints • Disinfect the spatula according to manufacturer's instructions. Some disinfectants may corrode metal or break down plastic. • The spatula should always be disinfected before and after use with a patient.

Flexible Mixing Spatula: Cement Spatula

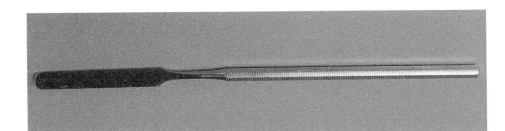

Use ▶ • To mix dental materials

◀▌▶ Special Notes/Helpful Hints • Ensure all residual dental materials have been removed from the spatula before sterilization. Bacteria can be present under the mixed material and live through a sterilization cycle, contributing to cross-contamination.

■ **MATERIAL**   Disposable Perforated Full-Arch Impression Trays

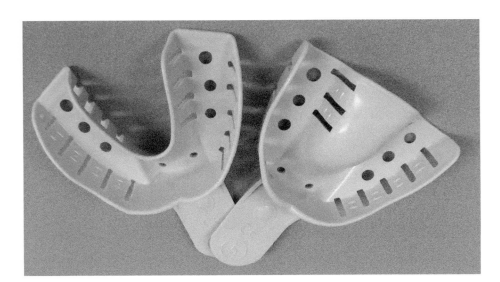

Use ▶ • To take intraoral impressions of the entire upper arch or lower arch with a variety of impression materials

◀▶ Special Notes/Helpful Hints • The impression tray has perforations, which allow the impression material to flow through the openings and lock into place. This action prevents the need for tray adhesive. • The impression tray is made of plastic and is considered to be disposable. The impression tray should be used with only one patient. • The impression tray can be used more than once in a single visit on the same patient if the quality of the impression is poor and the impression needs to be retaken. • When the impression has been determined to be of good quality, the impression should be poured. The impression tray should be thrown away after the model has been separated from the impression. • Attempting to sterilize plastic impression trays can cause the plastic to become porous; this allows bacteria to survive in the pores of the plastic, and cross-contamination can occur.

■ **MATERIAL** # Disposable Perforated Quadrant and Anterior Impression Trays

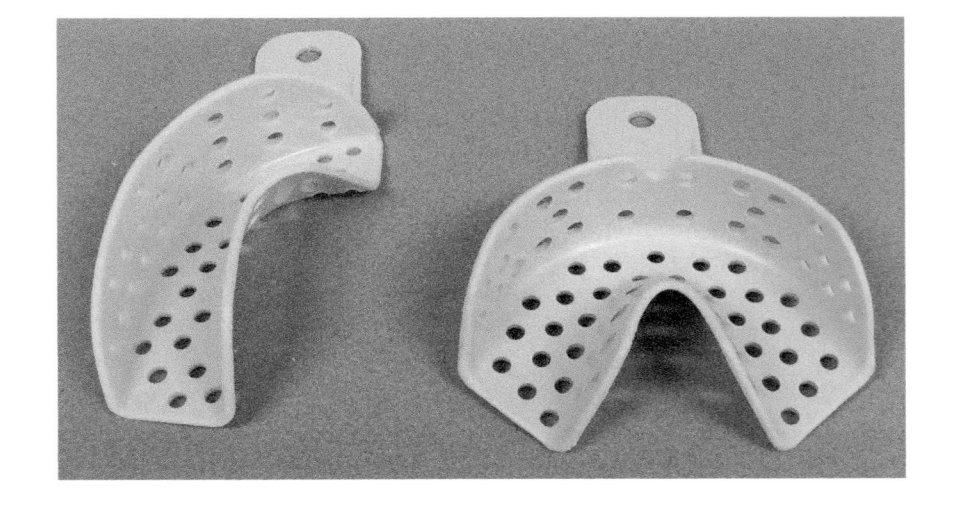

Use ▶ • To take intraoral impressions of one fourth of the upper arch or lower arch or the upper or lower anterior region of the dentition.

◀▌▶ Special Notes/Helpful Hints • The impression tray has perforations, which allow the impression material to flow through the openings and lock into place. This action eliminates the need for tray adhesive. • The impression tray is made of plastic, and the tray is considered to be disposable. The impression tray should be used with only one patient. • The impression tray can be used more than once in a single visit on the same patient if the quality of the impression is poor and the impression needs to be retaken. • When the impression has been determined to be of good quality, the impression should be poured. The impression tray should be thrown away after the model has been separated from the impression. • Attempting to sterilize plastic impression trays can cause the plastic to become porous; this allows bacteria to survive in the pores of the plastic, and cross-contamination can occur.

MATERIAL ■   Reusable Perforated Metal Impression Trays

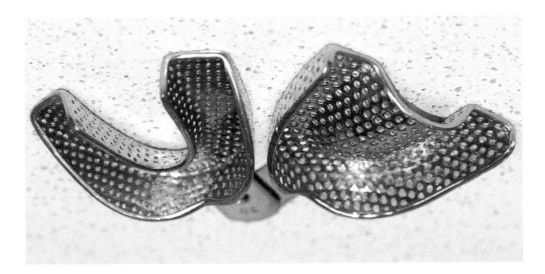

Use ▶ • To take intraoral impressions with a variety of impression materials

◀▣▷ Special Notes/Helpful Hints • The impression tray has perforations, which allow the impression material to flow through the openings and lock into place. This action eliminates the need for tray adhesive. • Metal impression trays must be cleaned thoroughly to ensure all residual impression material and gypsum have been removed before sterilization. Any residual material can harbor bacteria, resulting in cross-contamination. • Sterilize the impression tray according to manufacturer's instructions.

■ **MATERIAL** Reusable Nonperforated Metal Impression Trays

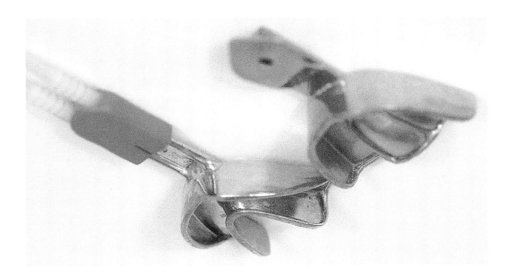

From Bird and Robinson, 2015.

• To take intraoral impressions with a variety of impression materials

◀▶ Special Notes/Helpful Hints • The impression tray does not have perforations, which means that the impression material cannot flow through the openings and lock into place. Tray adhesive should be used with nonperforated impression trays to assist in adherence of the impression material in the tray. • Metal impression trays must be cleaned thoroughly to ensure all residual impression material and gypsum have been removed before sterilization. Any residual material can harbor bacteria, resulting in cross-contamination. • Sterilize the impression tray according to manufacturer's instructions.

■ **MATERIAL** Triple Tray

From Boyd, 2015.

Use ► • To take final impressions for indirect restorations and bite registration simultaneously

◀▣▶ Special Notes/Helpful Hints • The triple tray is disposable and should be discarded when the final restoration has been successfully delivered to the patient.

Bite Registration Tray

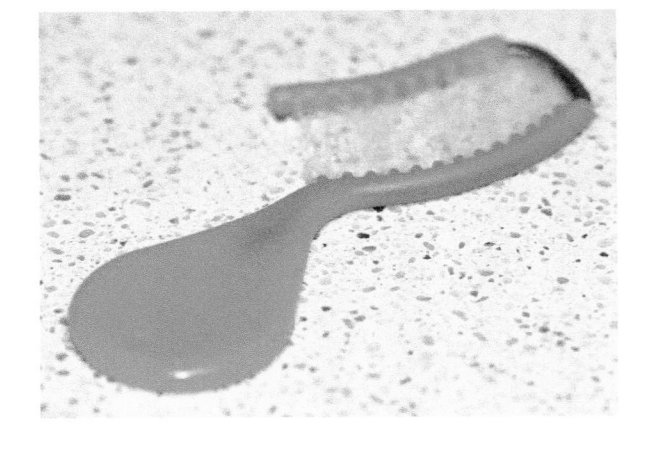

Use ▶ • To take a bite registration impression of the upper arch and lower arch simultaneously

◀▣▶ Special Notes/Helpful Hints • The bite registration tray is disposable and should be discarded when the final restoration has been successfully delivered to the patient.

■ **MATERIAL** Automixer

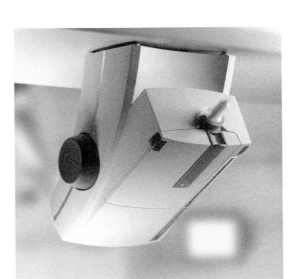

Courtesy 3 M ESPE Dental Products, Eagan, MN.

Use ▶ • To mix final impression material automatically

◀▶ Special Notes/Helpful Hints • Disinfect according to manufacturer's instructions. • Most manufacturers recommend leaving the mixing tip on the cartridge after use or replacing the mixing tip with the original cover to prevent the impression material from seeping out of the opening or becoming hard.

■ **MATERIAL**   Mixing Gun

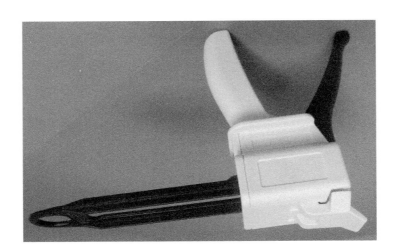

Uses ▶ • To mix final impression material
• To mix bite registration material
• To mix provisional crown material

◀▶ Special Notes/Helpful Hints • Disinfect according to manufacturer's instructions. • Most manufacturers recommend leaving the mixing tip on the cartridge after use or replacing the mixing tip with the original cover to prevent the material from seeping out of the opening or becoming hard.

MATERIAL Reversible Hydrocolloid Unit and Water-Cooled Impression Trays and Hose

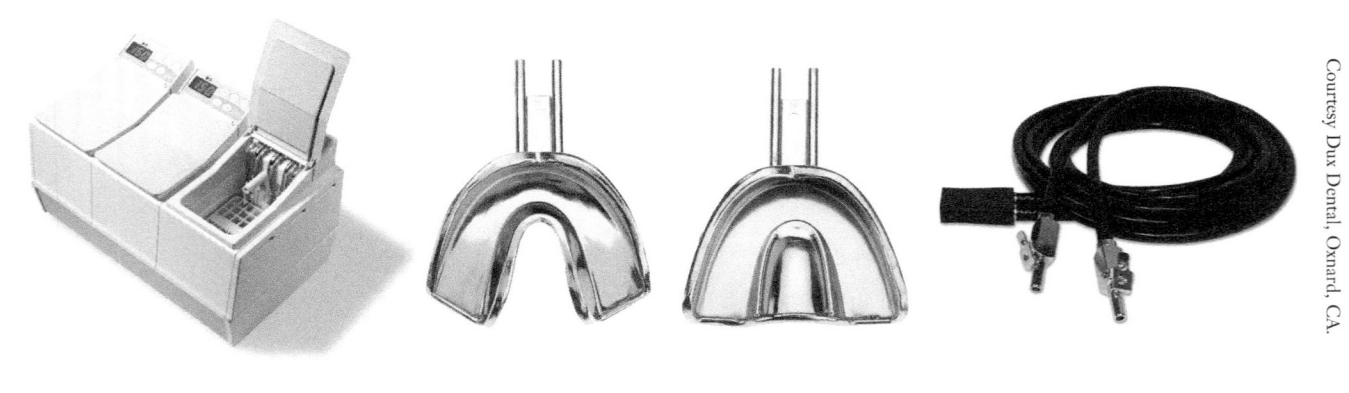

Uses ▶
- To store and heat reversible hydrocolloid impression material
- To take reversible hydrocolloid impressions

▶ Special Notes/Helpful Hints • The unit contains three chambers or baths for impression material. Fluids in the chambers should be changed between patients. • Disinfect according to manufacturer's instructions. • Metal impression trays must be cleaned thoroughly to ensure all residual impression material and gypsum have been removed before sterilization. Any residual material can harbor bacteria resulting in cross-contamination. • Sterilize impression tray according to manufacturer's instructions.

■ **MATERIAL**   Calcium Hydroxide Instrument

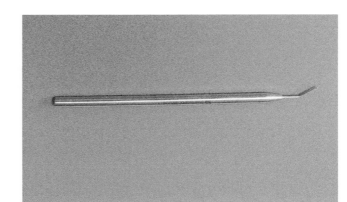

Use ▶ • To mix calcium hydroxide material

◀▮▶ Special Notes/Helpful Hints • Ensure all residual dental materials have been removed from the spatula prior to sterilization. Bacteria can be harbored under mixed material and live through a sterilization cycle, contributing to cross contamination.

MATERIAL

Dental Vibrator

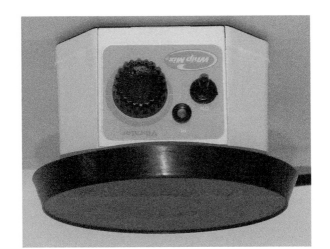

Uses ▶ • To vibrate air bubbles to the surface of mixed gypsum material
• To assist with flow of gypsum material into impression

◀▷ Special Notes/Helpful Hints • To maintain cleanliness of the machine, cover the vibrating platform with a plastic headrest cover or plastic bag. Using a cover assists in the cleaning and disinfecting process at the conclusion of use. • Disinfect the dental vibrator according to manufacturer's instructions.

■ MATERIAL Laboratory Knife

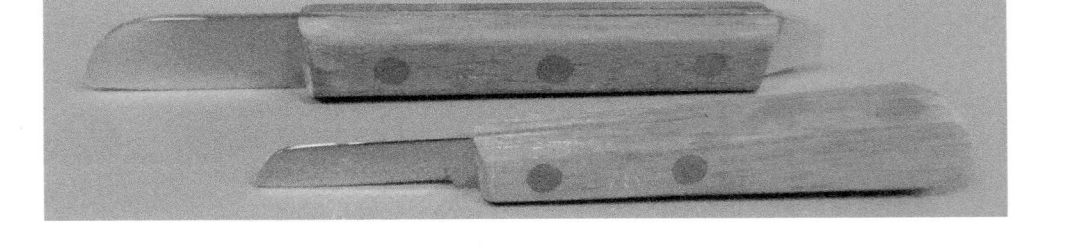

• To separate gypsum models from impressions
• To hand trim or shape models

▶ Special Notes/Helpful Hints • Residual material should be cleaned from the knife at the conclusion of use. • The knife must be sterilized if it becomes contaminated during use. • Sterilize the laboratory knife according to manufacturer's instructions.

■ **MATERIAL** Model Trimmer

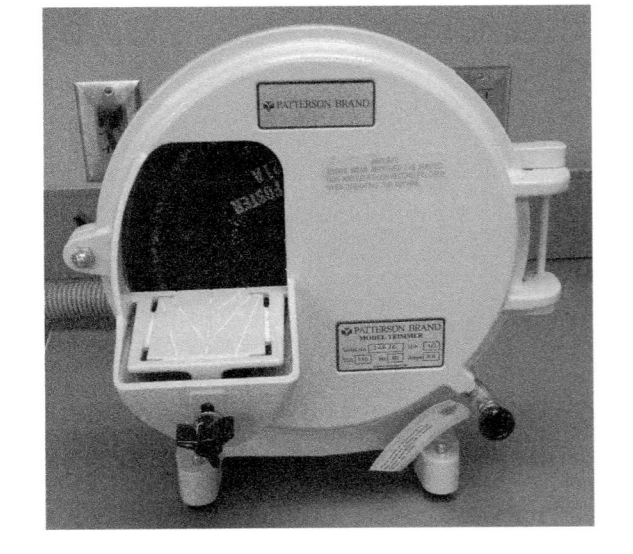

Use ▶ • To trim models made of gypsum products

◀▷ Special Notes/Helpful Hints • Personal protective equipment should be worn when using a model trimmer. At a minimum, mask and glasses should be worn. • Disinfect the model trimmer according to manufacturer's instructions.

■ **MATERIAL**   Dental Lathe

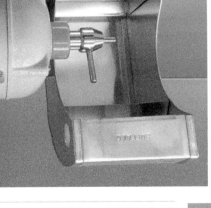

- To trim excess material off of models
- To trim excess material off of impression trays
- To polish a variety of appliances, such as orthodontic positioners, partial dentures, and full dentures

▶ Special Notes/Helpful Hints • Personal protective equipment should be worn when using a model trimmer. At a minimum, mask and glasses should be worn. • Disinfect the dental appliance being polished before polishing with a slurry of pumice. At the conclusion of use, the pumice should be discarded, and the rag wheel should be sterilized. • The same process should occur with the use of rouge. • Disinfect the dental lathe according to manufacturer's instructions.

MATERIAL Laboratory Handpiece

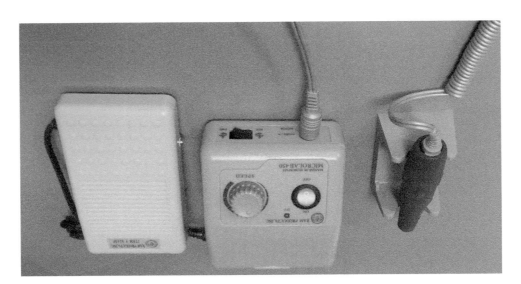

- To trim excess material off of models
- To trim excess material off of impression trays
- To smooth margins of a variety of appliances, such as bleaching trays, custom temporary crown forms, night guards, orthodontic positioners, and mouth guards

▶ Special Notes/Helpful Hints • Personal protective equipment should be worn when using a laboratory handpiece. At a minimum, mask and glasses should be worn. • Disinfect laboratory handpiece according to manufacturer's instructions. • Burs used in the laboratory handpiece can be sterilized.

■ **MATERIAL** Vacuum Former

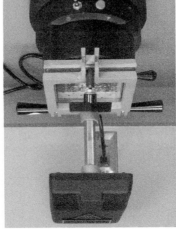

Use ▶ • To make a variety of appliances, such as bleaching trays, custom temporary crown forms, night guards, orthodontic positioners, and mouth guards

◀▮▷ Special Notes/Helpful Hints • Disinfect vacuum former according to manufacturer's instructions.

■ **MATERIAL** Amalgamator

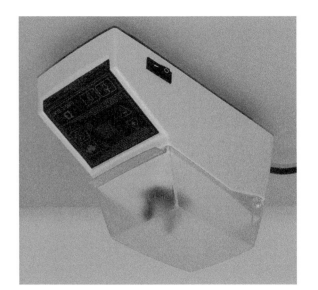

Uses ▶ • To triturate alloy and mercury into amalgam in a capsule
• To triturate other materials supplied in single-dose capsules that require mixing

◀▶ Special Notes/Helpful Hints • Set timer on amalgamator according to manufacturer's recommendation based on the material being triturated. • Disinfect amalgamator according to manufacturer's instructions.

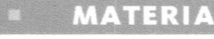 **MATERIAL** Curing Light

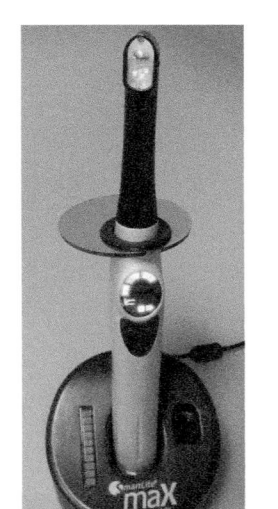

• To polymerize light-cured materials, such as bonding, composite, sealants, build-up material, and cements

Special Notes/Helpful Hints • Cover the tip of the curing light with a plastic protector to ensure dental materials do not adhere to surface of the light. • Disinfect curing light according to manufacturer's instructions. • Ensure that the curing light maintains a charge if the light is rechargeable.

Alcohol Burner

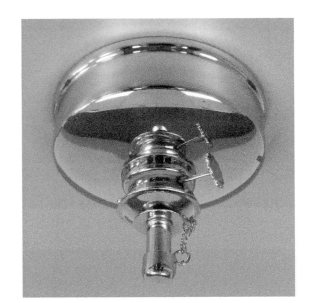

• To heat dental materials
• To smooth surfaces of appliances, such as whitening trays, orthodontic positioners, night guards, and mouth guards after being trimmed

◀▣▶ Special Notes/Helpful Hints • Denatured alcohol should be used in an alcohol burner. • Disinfect alcohol torch according to manufacturer's instructions.

■ **MATERIAL** ■ Glass Slab

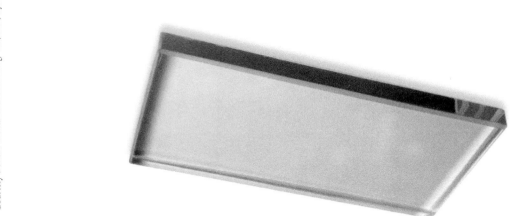

Courtesy Buffalo Dental Manufacturing Co., Inc., Syosset, NY.

Use ▶ • To mix different types of dental materials

◖▶ Special Notes/Helpful Hints • Sterilize glass slab according to manufacturer's instructions. • Store glass slabs in the refrigerator because most manufacturers recommend using a chilled slab to increase working time or dissipate heat as a result of an exothermic reaction. If a chilled slab is not needed, the slab can remain out in the open to become room temperature.

MATERIAL ■

Dappen Dish

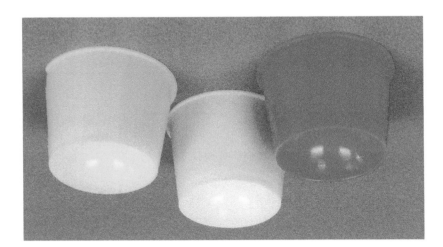

Uses ▶ • To mix different types of dental materials
• To store material while in use

▶ Special Notes/Helpful Hints • Reusable and disposable dappen dishes are available. • Disposable dappen dishes should be discarded after one use. • Reusable dappen dishes should be disinfected according to manufacturer's instructions.

MATERIAL Mixing Well

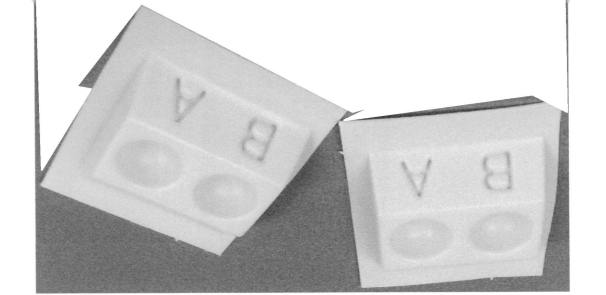

Uses ▶ • To mix different types of dental materials
• To store material while in use

◀▶ Special Notes/Helpful Hints • Reusable and disposable mixing wells are available. • Disposable mixing wells should be discarded after one use. • Reusable mixing wells should be disinfected according to manufacturer's instructions.

MATERIAL   Paper Mixing Pads

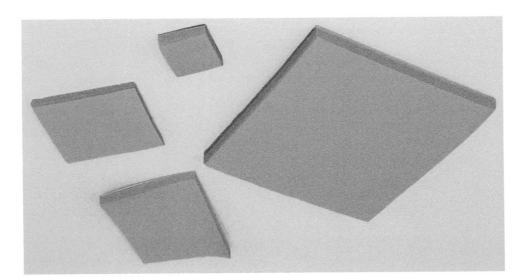

• To mix different types of dental materials

▶ Special Notes/Helpful Hints • Each paper is coated with wax or some other type of fluid-resistant material to prevent liquid from seeping through paper. • Paper pads come in a variety of sizes. • Manufacturers may require a special paper pad be used with their specific material or suggest a specific size pad according to the surface area needed to mix material. • To prevent cross-contamination with a paper mixing pad, one paper should be removed from the stack, or overgloves should be used. Never mix material on the entire stack with contaminated gloves. It is impossible to disinfect or sterilize the entire stack. If contamination occurs, the stack must be thrown out.

■ **MATERIAL** Mandrel

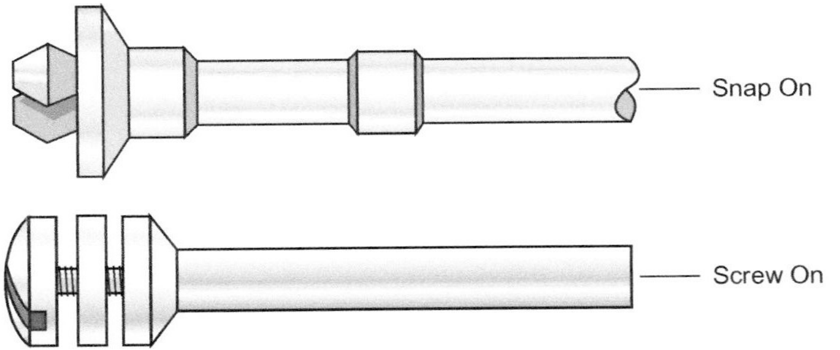

From Boyd, 2015.

Snap On

Screw On

Use ▶ • To attach discs containing abrasives for finishing and polishing a tooth structure or appliances

◀▮▶ Special Notes/Helpful Hints • A mandrel is inserted into and secured in a handpiece. • The mandrel must be sterilized after use.

MATERIAL Disposable Applicator (Microbrush)

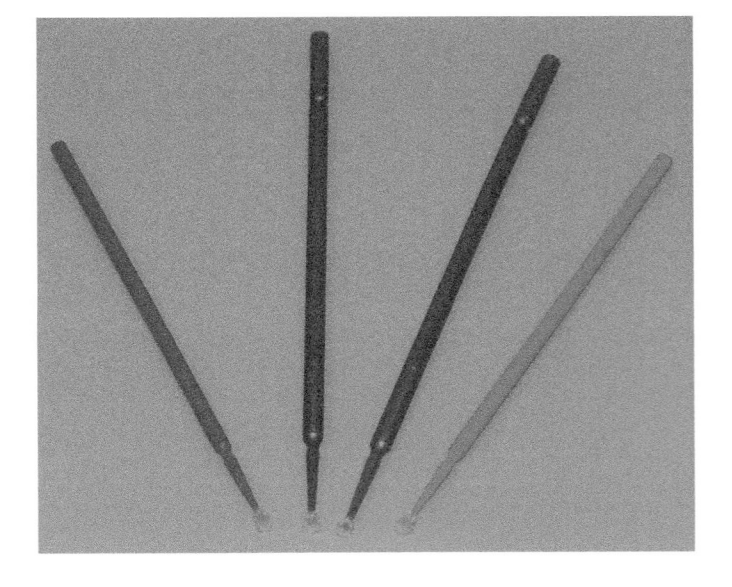

Uses ▶ • To apply materials to the tooth surface
• To spread material across the tooth surface when air cannot be used

◀▶ Special Notes/Helpful Hints • Disposable applicators come in a variety of sizes. • The tip of the applicator can usually be bent to accommodate hard-to-reach places.

■ **MATERIAL** ■ Soft Guard Material

• To fabricate an appliance to deliver dental material intraorally
• To protect the tooth structure from trauma

Special Notes/Helpful Hints • Soft guard material comes in a variety of thicknesses and colors. • This material is used most frequently to make whitening trays and sports guards; however, it can be used as a night guard or for delivery of home fluoride treatments.

Liners and Bases

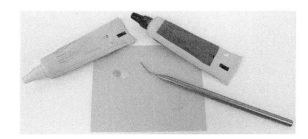

MATERIAL   Varnish

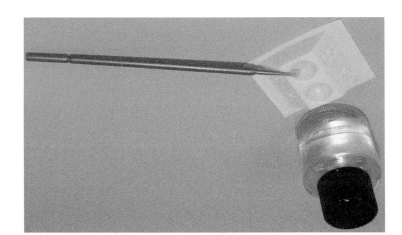

How Supplied ▶ Liquid

Composition ▶ Resin dissolved in solvent

• Varnish
• Dappen dish

• Disposable applicator (Microbrush)
• Restorative instruments

Directions ▶ 1. Prepare tooth for restoration.
2. Dispense varnish into Dappen dish when ready to use. Do not dispense material early because it will evaporate.
3. Using disposable applicator, paint varnish on the inside of the cavity preparation.
4. Allow to dry.
5. Place restorative material.

◀▶ Special Notes/Helpful Hints • Varnish leaves a thin layer of material that is used to protect the pulp. • Varnish is also used to provide a thin layer over the surface of glass ionomer when it has been initially placed because the material takes 24 hours to set fully.

■ **MATERIAL** Calcium Hydroxide

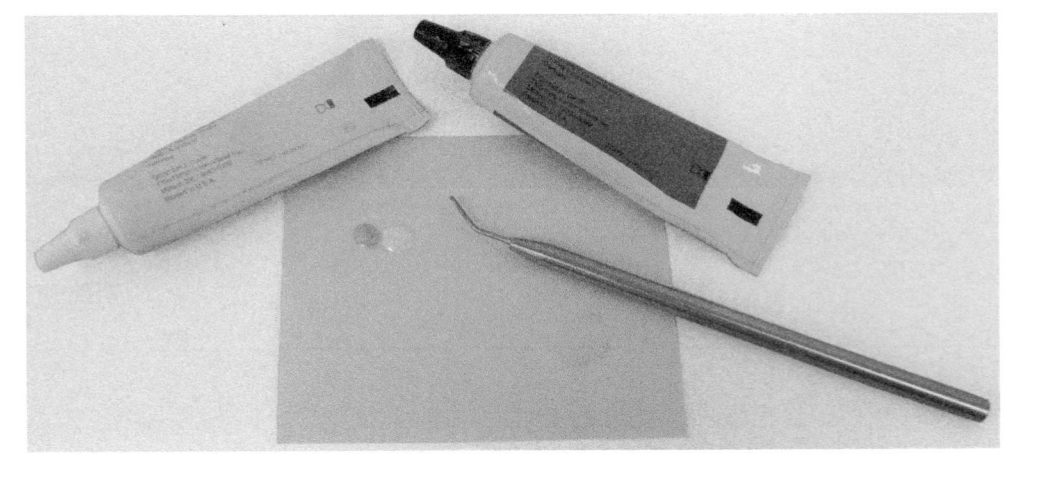

How Supplied ▶ Two pastes in tubes

Composition ▶ Base paste—calcium tungstate, calcium phosphate, and zinc oxide in glycol salicylate

• Calcium hydroxide material   • Calcium hydroxide instrument
• Mixing pad   • Restorative instruments

Directions ▶ 1. Dispense two pastes in equal amounts on a paper mixing pad.
2. Using calcium hydroxide instrument, swirl together pastes until a homogeneous paste is obtained.
3. Using a piece of gauze, clean off the tip of calcium hydroxide instrument.
4. Use the calcium hydroxide instrument to gather a small amount of the material on the tip of the instrument, and place the material in the area of the prepared tooth cavity, where needed.

◀▶ Special Notes/Helpful Hints • Calcium hydroxide is used for direct and indirect pulp capping and as a protective barrier beneath composite restorations. • The material is very easy to use because its setting reaction is accelerated with water. • Moisture in dentin causes the material to set within seconds. • Calcium hydroxide is a low-strength base.

■ **MATERIAL**

Glass Ionomer: Powder and Liquid

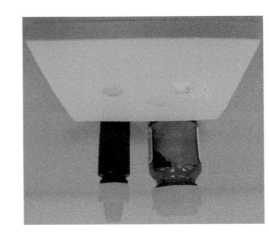

How Supplied ▶ Powder and liquid

Premeasured single-dose capsules

Composition ▶ Powder—aluminosilicate glass

Armamentarium ▶
- Glass ionomer cement
- Wax-coated mixing pad (when pastes or powder and liquid systems are used)
- Cement spatula
- Restorative instruments

Directions ▶ For powder and liquid systems:

1. Measure powder using scoop provided by manufacturer, and dispense onto mixing pad.
2. Dispense liquid as droplets onto the mixing pad.
3. Force powder into liquid, and mix quickly to ensure a mixing time of 30 to 45 seconds is not exceeded.
4. Use side of spatula to scrape up mixed material.
5. Dry the area where material is to be placed, and then place material into the prepared tooth.

▶ Special Notes/Helpful Hints • The manufacturer's recommended powder-to-liquid ratios should be followed. • Some glass ionomer restorative materials used for liners and bases require polymerization with the curing light. • Glass ionomer releases fluoride and is recommended for use on patients with a high risk of caries.

MATERIAL ■ Glass Ionomer: Single-Dose Capsules

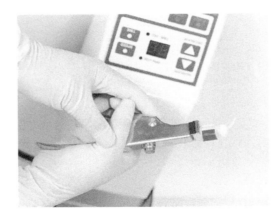

From Hatrick, Eakle, and Bird, 2011.

◄ **How Supplied**
Powder and liquid
Premeasured single-dose capsules

◄ **Composition**
Powder—aluminosilicate glass
Liquid—polymers and copolymers of acrylic acid

Armamentarium ▶
- Glass ionomer cement single-dose capsule
- Amalgamator
- Dispensing syringe
- Restorative instruments

Directions ▶ For single-dose capsule systems:

1. Activate capsule, if indicated by manufacturer.
2. Place capsule in amalgamator, and triturate capsule for the amount of time indicated by manufacturer.
3. Remove capsule from the amalgamator, and immediately place capsule into the dispenser provided by the manufacturer.
4. Dry the area where material is to be placed.
5. Advance the mixed material to the tip of the capsule, and dispense material into prepared tooth with dispenser.

⬛▷ Special Notes/Helpful Hints • The manufacturer's recommended powder-to-liquid ratios should be followed. • Glass ionomer releases fluoride and is recommended for use on patients with a high risk of caries.

MATERIAL

Resin-Modified Calcium Silicate: Powder and Liquid

How Supplied ► Powder and liquid

Premeasured single-dose capsules

Composition ► Powder—radiopaque, fluoroaluminosilicate glass

• Resin-modified glass ionomer
• Wax-coated mixing pad (when pastes or powder and liquid systems are used)
• Cement spatula
• Curing light
• Restorative instruments

Directions ▶ For powder and liquid:

1. Fluff powder by shaking bottle gently.
2. Measure powder using scoop provided by manufacturer, and dispense onto mixing pad.
3. Holding the vial of liquid vertically, dispense liquid as droplets.
4. Force powder into liquid, and mix quickly to ensure a mixing time of 30 to 45 seconds is not exceeded.
5. Use side of spatula to scrape up mixed material.
6. Dry area where material is to be placed, and then place material into prepared tooth.
7. Polymerize with curing light.

▶ Special Notes/Helpful Hints • Resin-modified glass ionomer should have a mousselike consistency when mixed. • Working time is usually 2.5 minutes. Refer to manufacturer's instructions for recommendations. • The manufacturer's recommended powder-to-liquid ratios should be followed.

■ **MATERIAL**

Resin-Modified Calcium Silicate: Single-Dose Capsule

How Supplied ◂ Powder and liquid

Premeasured single-dose capsules

Composition ◂ Powder—radiopaque, fluoroaluminosilicate glass

Liquid—monomers, polyacids, and water

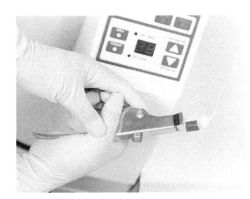

From Hatrick, Eakle, and Bird, 2011.

• Resin-modified glass ionomer single-dose capsule
• Amalgamator
• Dispensing syringe
• Curing light
• Restorative instruments

Directions ▶ For single-dose capsule:

1. Etch or prime tooth according to manufacturer's instruction for the particular product being used.
2. Dry area where base is to be placed, and maintain isolation.
3. Activate glass ionomer restorative material capsule by placing the capsule in the capsule activator and depressing the lever.
4. Place the capsule in the amalgamator, and mix for the time indicated in the manufacturer's instructions.
5. Place capsule in dispensing gun, and place material into the prepared tooth structure.
6. Contour material into the proper shape with composite placement instrument or plastic instrument.
7. Polymerize material with curing light.

◀▶ Special Notes/Helpful Hints • Resin-modified glass ionomer should have a mousselike consistency when mixed. • Working time is usually 2.5 minutes. Refer to manufacturer's instructions for recommendations.

Bonding Agents

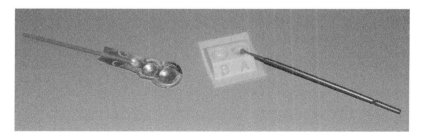

■ **MATERIAL** Etchant

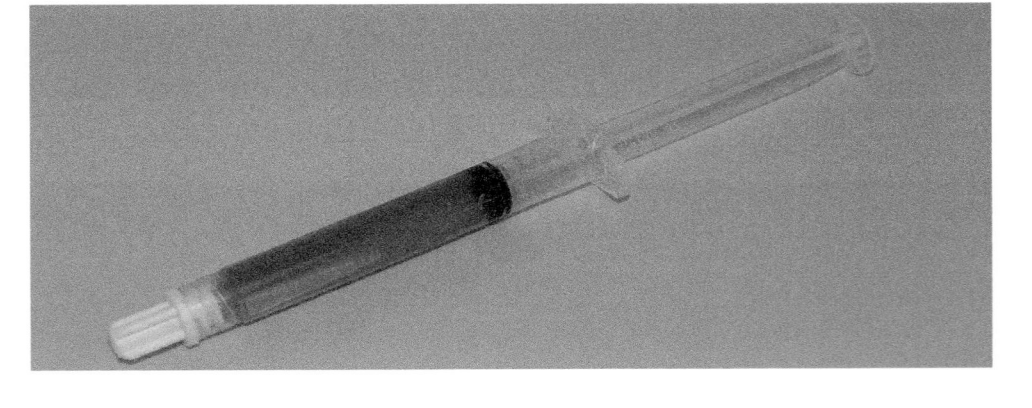

How Supplied ▶ Gel

Composition ▶ 37% Orthophosphoric acid

- Etchant
- Restorative instruments

1. Coat tooth surface to be restored with etchant (37% orthophosphoric acid gel)
2. Allow etchant to remain on tooth surface for amount of time indicated by manufacturer.
3. Rinse etchant from tooth surface for amount of time indicated by manufacturer.
4. Dry area for amount of time indicated by manufacturer.
5. Tooth surface will appear chalky white if tooth has been etched for the appropriate amount of time.
6. Place bonding or restorative material on tooth surface, depending on procedure being completed.

▐▶ Special Notes/Helpful Hints • Etch time must be extended for primary teeth due to the irregularly shaped enamel rods. • Etch time must be extended for tooth surfaces recently treated with fluoride. • Variances occur in the percentage of orthophosphoric acid, depending on the manufacturer of the etchant. If an etchant has a lower percentage of orthophosphoric acid the etch time will increase, while a higher percentage of orthophosphoric acid will decrease the etch time.

MATERIAL Total Etch "Three-Step" Bonding Agent

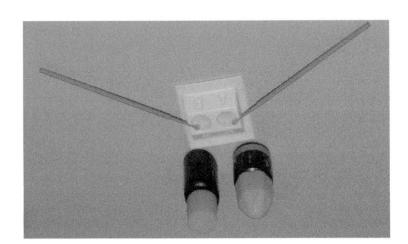

How Supplied ◄ Liquid

Composition ◄ Dimethacrylate, silanated colloidal silica

Armamentarium ▶
- Etchant
- Bonding system
- Disposable applicator (Microbrush)
- Dappen dish or mixing dish
- Restorative instruments
- Curing light

Directions ▶
1. Etch prepared tooth structure with 37% phosphoric acid gel.
2. Rinse tooth with water, ensuring all etchant has been removed, and dry surface gently with a stream of compressed air.
3. Apply primer to etched tooth surface with Microbrush. Blow tooth surface gently with compressed air, if indicated by the manufacturer.
4. Apply bonding to tooth surface with Microbrush. Thin material with a light puff of compressed air, and then light cure.
5. Place restorative material in prepared tooth structure.

◀▶ Special Notes/Helpful Hints Bonding agents usually begin to polymerize when exposed to ambient light. Using a mixing dish with a covering can protect the material while each step is being completed. • Ensure the compressed air is not contaminated with water prior to drying tooth surface or thinning materials. This may be accomplished by depressing the air button on the air/water syringe prior to use intraorally.

MATERIAL

Total Etch "Two-Step" Bonding Agent

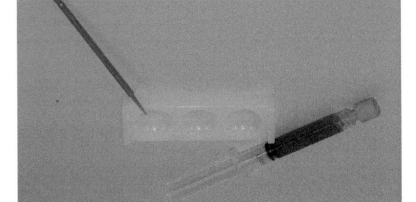

How Supplied ◄ Liquid

Composition ◄ Dimethacrylate silanated colloidal silica

• Etchant
• Bonding system
• Disposable applicator (Microbrush)
• Dappen dish or mixing dish
• Restorative instruments
• Curing light

Directions ▶ 1. Etch prepared tooth structure with 37% phosphoric acid gel.
2. Rinse tooth with water, ensuring all etchant has been removed, and dry surface gently with a stream of compressed air.
3. Apply bonding generously to tooth surface with Microbrush.
4. Allow bonding to set for 15 seconds.
5. Dry with light compressed air until no movement of bonding agent (liquid) can be seen.
6. Place restorative material in prepared tooth structure.

▶ Special Notes/Helpful Hints Bonding agents usually begin to polymerize when exposed to ambient light. Using a mixing dish with a covering can protect the material while each step is being completed. • Ensure the compressed air is not contaminated with water prior to drying tooth surface or thinning materials. This may be accomplished by depressing the air button on the air/water syringe prior to use intraorally.

■ MATERIAL

Self-Etch "One Bottle" Bonding Agent

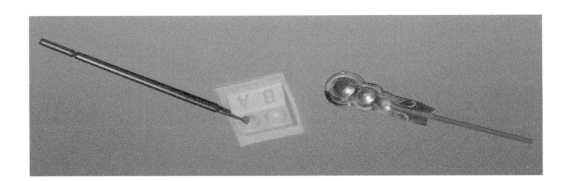

How Supplied ◄ Liquid in a single-dose unit

Composition ◄ Dimethacrylate, phosphoric acid, and other additives

- Bonding system
- Disposable applicator
- Curing light
- Restorative instruments

Directions ▶

1. Remove loose debris from tooth preparation by spraying water on the surface. If the tooth has not been prepared for a restoration, clean untreated tooth structure with a rubber cup and slurry of pumice and water.
2. Use two to three brief puffs of compressed air to dry cavity. Do not overdry cavity because it may cause sensitivity.
3. If mixing is required, mix material according to manufacturer's instructions.
4. Brush material onto the entire cavity, and massage it in by applying pressure. Longer massaging times may be required for larger surfaces.
5. Use a gentle stream of compressed air to dry the adhesive thoroughly to a thin film.
6. Rewet the disposable applicator tip with adhesive, and apply a second coat. This coat does not need to be massaged in.
7. Use a gentle stream of compressed air to dry the adhesive thoroughly to a thin film.
8. Polymerize the material with a curing light.
9. Place restorative material in prepared tooth structure.

▶ Special Notes/Helpful Hints • Bonding agents usually bond more efficiently to a moist surface rather than one that is dry or overly wet. • Manufacturers' instructions vary greatly for bonding agents. Follow the specific manufacturer's instructions carefully for the best results. • Overdrying the preparation before application of the adhesive has been known to cause sensitivity. • Ensure the compressed air is not contaminated with water prior to drying tooth surface or thinning materials. This may be accomplished by depressing the air button on the air/water syringe prior to use intraorally.

◼ **MATERIAL** Self-Etch "Two Bottle" Bonding Agent

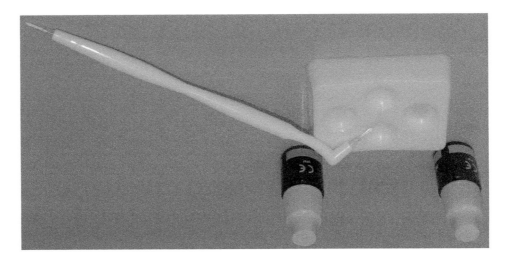

How Supplied ◀ Liquid in two bottles

Composition ◀ Dimethacrylate, phosphoric acid, and other additives

Armamentarium ▶
- Bonding system
- Disposable applicator(s)
- Restorative instruments

Directions ▶
1. Remove loose debris from tooth preparation by spraying water on the surface. If tooth has not been prepared for a restoration, clean untreated tooth structure with rubber cup and a slurry of pumice and water.
2. Use 2-3 brief puffs of compressed air to dry cavity. Do not overdry cavity as it may cause sensitivity.
3. Mix material according to manufacturer's instructions if mixing is required
4. Brush acid primer onto the entire cavity with disposable applicator.
5. Use a gentle stream of compressed air to thin primer.
6. Use second disposable applicator tip to apply bonding resin to tooth surface.
7. Use a gentle stream of compressed air to thoroughly dry the adhesive to a thin film.
8. Polymerize the material with a curing light only if indicated by manufacturer's instructions.
9. Place restorative material in prepared tooth structure.

◀▶ Special Notes/Helpful Hints • Bonding agents usually bond more efficiently to a moist surface rather than one that is dry or overly wet. • Manufacturer's instructions vary greatly for bonding agents. Be sure to follow the manufacturer's instructions carefully for the best results. • Overdrying the preparation prior to the application of the adhesive has been known to cause sensitivity. • Ensure the compressed air is not contaminated with water prior to drying tooth surface or thinning materials. This may be accomplished by depressing the air button on the air/water syringe prior to use intraorally.

4

Amalgam Restorative Materials

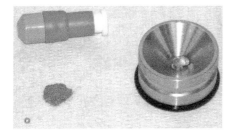

Admix High-Copper Dental Amalgam

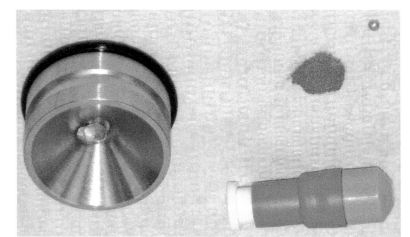

How Supplied ◂ Capsules

Composition ◂ Silver, copper, tin, and liquid mercury

• Amalgam capsules
• Amalgamator
• Amalgam well
• Amalgam carrier
• Restorative instruments
• Cotton roll
• Tofflemire, matrix band, and wedge (if restoration is a class II)

Directions ▶ 1. Activate amalgam restorative material capsule by squeezing the two ends of capsule together, if indicated by manufacturer.
2. Place capsule in amalgamator and triturate for the time indicated in manufacturer's instructions.
3. Dry area where restoration is to be placed, and maintain isolation.
4. Place mixed amalgam in amalgam well.
5. Load amalgam carrier with mixed amalgam and carry amalgam to prepared tooth structure.
6. Place material into prepared tooth structure.
7. Using a condenser, press and condense amalgam into prepared tooth structure.
8. Continue to load prepared tooth with amalgam while condensing the material into prepared tooth structure.

◄ Cont'd Directions

9. When prepared tooth structure has been overfilled with amalgam and all the material has been condensed or packed into the prepared tooth structure, begin carving and shaping of restoration.

10. Burnish the outer surface of restoration with a football or ball burnisher.

11. Carve away excess material with a Hollenback carver, Wedelstadt chisel, or other instrument of choice.

12. Burnish amalgam again with football or ball burnisher, or use an acorn burnisher to place grooves into the surface of the amalgam.

13. Wet a cotton roll and rub cotton roll over surface of amalgam to remove any excess material remaining from carving.

If the prepared tooth is a class II preparation, a matrix band and wedge will need to be used to maintain the shape of the restoration during placement. The matrix band should be placed before the activation or trituration of amalgam.

Special Notes/Helpful Hints • The first high-copper amalgam was called Dispersalloy. • To be considered a high-copper amalgam, the mixture must contain 10% to 30% copper. • "Blended," "admixed," or "dispersion" alloys are a mixture of two kinds of particles. A clinician is unable to identify by sight if the particles in an amalgam are blended, admixed, or dispersion without the use of a microscope. • Amalgam does not fully set-up until 24 hours after placement. • Final polishing or adjustment should not occur for a minimum of 24 hours.

Spherical High-Copper Dental Amalgam

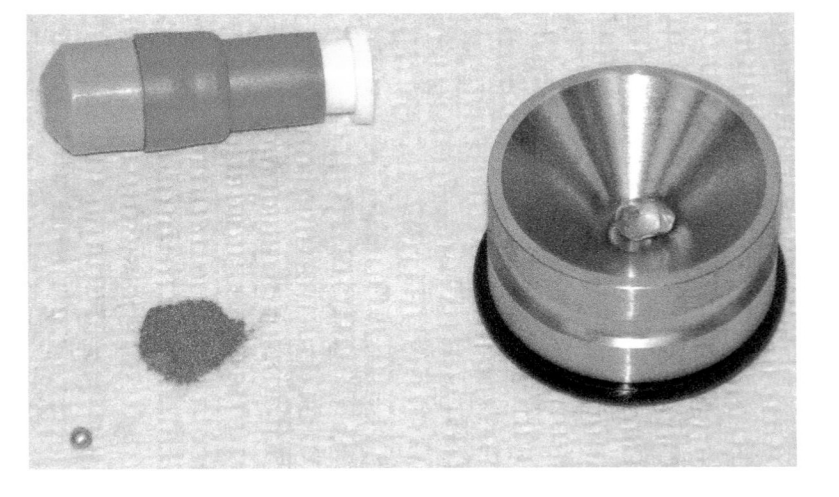

How Supplied ▶ Capsules

Composition ▶ Silver, copper, tin, and liquid mercury

Armamentarium ▶
- Amalgam capsule
- Amalgamator
- Amalgam well
- Amalgam carrier
- Restorative instruments
- Cotton roll
- Tofflemire, matrix band, and wedge (if restoration is a class II)

Directions ▶
1. Activate amalgam restorative material capsule by squeezing the two ends of capsule together, if indicated by manufacturer.
2. Place capsule in the amalgamator and triturate for the time indicated in manufacturer's instructions.
3. Dry area where restoration is to be placed, and maintain isolation.
4. Place mixed amalgam in amalgam well.
5. Load amalgam carrier with mixed amalgam and carry amalgam to prepared tooth structure.
6. Place material into prepared tooth structure.

Cont'd Directions ►

7. Using a condenser press, condense amalgam into prepared tooth structure.

8. Continue to load prepared tooth with amalgam while condensing material into prepared tooth structure.

9. When prepared tooth structure has been overfilled with amalgam and all the material has been condensed or packed into the prepared tooth structure, begin carving and shaping of restoration.

10. Burnish the outer surface of the restoration with a football or ball burnisher.

11. Carve away excess material with a Hollenback carver, Wedelstadt chisel, or other instrument of choice.

12. Burnish amalgam again with football or ball burnisher, or use an acorn burnisher to place grooves into the surface of the amalgam.

13. Wet a cotton roll and rub cotton roll over surface of amalgam to remove any excess material remaining from carving.

If the prepared tooth is a class II preparation, a matrix band and wedge will need to be used to maintain the shape of the restoration during placement. The matrix band should be placed before activation or trituration of amalgam.

▶ **Special Notes/Helpful Hints** • Spherical high-copper dental amalgam has a single composition, meaning only one shape of particle is present. A clinician is unable to identify by sight if the particles in an amalgam are spherical without the use of a microscope. • The first single-composition spherical dental amalgam was Tytin. • To be considered a high-copper amalgam, the mixture must contain 10% to 30% copper. • Spherical high-copper dental amalgam has a mushy feel when it is freshly triturated and it is easy to condense because of its single composition. • Amalgam does not fully set-up until 24 hours after placement. • Final polishing or adjustment should not occur for a minimum of 24 hours.

5

Resin Restorative Materials

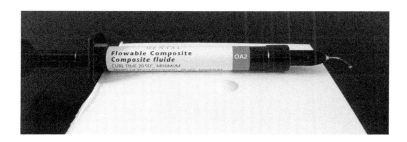

■ **MATERIAL** Macrofilled Composite

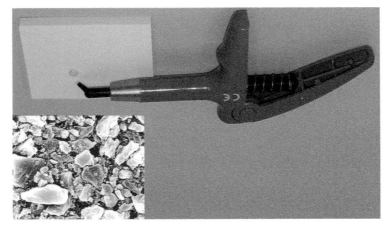

Inset photo from Freedman, 2012.

◄ **How Supplied** Syringes or single-use cartridge

◄ **Composition** Composite resin and silica

Armamentarium ▶
- Composite
- Etchant
- Bonding system

- Curing light
- Restorative instruments
- Composite placement instrument

Directions ▶
1. Etch tooth surface with 37% orthophosphoric acid.
2. Rinse lightly and dry.
3. Prepare etched tooth surface with primer and bonding agent.
4. Place composite material in desired location and shape with composite placement instrument.
5. Polymerize with curing light.
6. Adjust and finish material.

▶ Special Notes/Helpful Hints • A clinician is unable to identify by sight if a composite is macrofilled without the use of a microscope. • Macrofilled composites have large filler particles, which result in a restoration that feels rough to a dental explorer and can appear rough to the eye. The likelihood of plaque accumulation and stain is greater. • This material is used most frequently by orthodontists to bond brackets or other orthodontic appliances.

■ **MATERIAL** Microfilled Composite

How Supplied ◄ Syringes or single-use cartridge

Composition ◄ Composite resin and finely ground silica

Armamentarium ▶
- Composite
- Etchant
- Bonding system
- Curing light
- Restorative instruments
- Composite placement instrument

Directions ▶
1. Etch tooth surface with 37% orthophosphoric acid.
2. Rinse lightly and dry.
3. Prepare etched tooth surface with primer and bonding agent.
4. Place composite material in desired location and shape with composite placement instrument.
5. Polymerize with curing light.
6. Adjust and finish material.

◀▶ Special Notes/Helpful Hints • A clinician is unable to identify by sight if a composite is microfilled without the use of a microscope. • Microfilled composites have small filler particles, which results in a low modulus of elasticity. • Because of their high luster, microfilled composites are most frequently used for class V restorations or as the top layer on an anterior restoration. • Microfilled composites can be polished to a high luster to look like enamel.

■ **MATERIAL** Hybrid Composite

Inset photo from Freedman, 2012.

◂ **How Supplied** Syringes or single-use cartridge

◂ **Composition** Composite resin and silica (composition is a combination of microparticles and macroparticles)

- Composite
- Etchant
- Bonding system
- Curing light
- Restorative instruments
- Composite placement instrument

Directions ▶
1. Etch tooth surface with 37% orthophosphoric acid.
2. Rinse lightly and dry.
3. Prepare etched tooth surface with primer and bonding agent.
4. Place composite material in desired location and shape with plastic instrument.
5. Polymerize with curing light.
6. Adjust and finish material.

◀▶ Special Notes/Helpful Hints • Hybrid composites have different-sized filler particles, which result in a strong material that polishes well. • A clinician is unable to identify by sight if a composite is a hybrid composite without the use of a microscope. • Because of their strength and abrasion resistance, hybrid composites are acceptable for class I and II restorations.

■ **MATERIAL** ▬ Improved Hybrid Composite

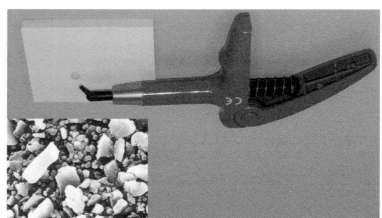

Inset photo from Freedman, 2012.

How Supplied ▸ Single-use cartridge

Composition ▸ Composite resin and silica

- Composite
- Composite gun
- Etchant
- Bonding system

- Curing light
- Restorative instruments
- Composite placement instrument

Directions ▶
1. Etch tooth surface with 37% orthophosphoric acid.
2. Rinse lightly and dry.
3. Prepare etched tooth surface with primer and bonding agent.
4. Place composite material in desired location and shape with composite placement instrument.
5. Polymerize with curing light.
6. Adjust and finish material.

◀▶ Special Notes/Helpful Hints • The average particle size in improved hybrid composites is decreased compared with hybrid composites, and nano-sized particles have been added. • Nano-sized particles are approximately 100 times smaller than the thickness of human hair. The results are slight improvements in strength and polymerization shrinkage and a smooth surface, which allows the material to be polished to a smooth and lustrous finish. • A clinician is unable to identify by sight if a composite is an improved hybrid composite without the use of a microscope.

■ **MATERIAL** — Flowable Composite

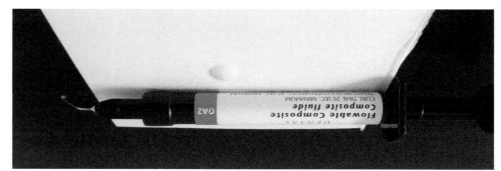

How Supplied ◀ Syringe or single-use cartridge

Composition ◀ Organic resin matrix, inorganic filler, and silane

• Composite material
• Etchant
• Bonding system

• Curing light
• Restorative instruments
• Composite placement instrument

Directions ▶ 1. Etch tooth surface with 37% orthophosphoric acid.
2. Rinse lightly and dry.
3. Prepare etched tooth surface with primer and bonding agent.
4. Depending on how composite is supplied, place composite cartridge in dispensing gun, or place Luer-Lok applicator tips on syringe.
5. Place composite in desired location and shape with composite placement instrument or tip of Shepard's hook explorer.
6. Polymerize with curing light.
7. Adjust and finish flowable composite material, or place hybrid material.

◀▶ Special Notes/Helpful Hints • The filler content of flowable composite has been decreased to allow the material to be less viscous and to flow. A weaker, less abrasion-resistant material is the result. • Flowable composites are typically used as the initial increment of a composite restoration, which is then covered with a hybrid material.

MATERIAL Resin-Modified Glass Ionomer: Light-Activated or Hybrid Ionomers

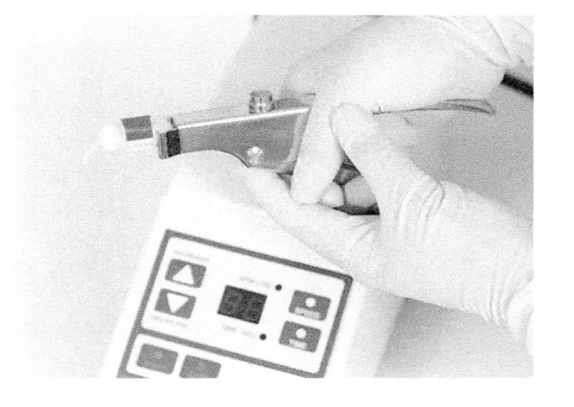

From Hatrick, Eakle, and Bird, 2011.

How Supplied ▶ Capsule

Composition ▶ Powder—aluminosilicate glass
Liquid—monomers, polyacrylic acid, and water

Armamentarium ▶ • Glass ionomer restorative material
• Capsule activator
• Amalgamator
• Dispensing gun
• Restorative instruments
• Composite placement instrument

Directions ▶ 1. Etch or prime tooth according to manufacturer's instructions for the particular product being used.
2. Dry area where restoration is to be placed, and maintain isolation.
3. Activate glass ionomer restorative material capsule by placing capsule in capsule activator and depressing lever.

Cont'd Directions ▶

4. Place capsule in amalgamator and mix for the time indicated in manufacturer's instructions.
5. Place capsule in dispensing gun and dispense material into prepared tooth structure.
6. Contour material into proper shape with a composite placement instrument or plastic instrument.
7. Polymerize material with curing light.
8. Adjust and finish material.

▶ Special Notes/Helpful Hints • Resin-modified glass ionomers are a little stronger and tougher than chemically-activated glass ionomers. • Resin-modified glass ionomer releases more fluoride than composite and compomers but less than traditional glass ionomer. The material releases fluoride over time, but the fluoride released by the material decreases over time. The fluoride in the resin-modified glass ionomer can be recharged with topical fluoride application. • This material is recommended for patients with a high risk of caries. • Resin-modified glass ionomer is more esthetically pleasing than traditional glass ionomer because of the addition of resin. • Most clinicians believe bonding must be used with resin-modified glass ionomer because of the resin content, but bonding is contraindicated. The bonding prevents the release of fluoride from the material to the tooth.

■ **MATERIAL**

Glass Ionomer Restorative Materials (Chemically Activated): Powder and Liquid

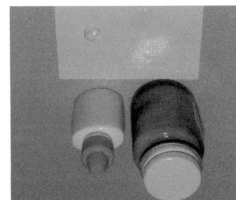

How Supplied ◀ Powder and liquid or single-dose capsules

Composition ◀ Powder—aluminosilicate glass

• Glass ionomer restorative material
• Wax-coated mixing pad
• Flexible mixing spatula
• Restorative instruments

Directions ▶ For powder and liquid systems:

1. Tumble bottle of powder gently.
2. Measure powder using scoop provided by manufacturer, and dispense onto mixing pad.
3. Dispense liquid as droplets onto mixing pad.
4. Force powder into liquid, and mix quickly to ensure a mixing time of 30 to 45 seconds is not exceeded; a viscous material with the consistency of cake icing should result.
5. Use the side of the spatula to scrape up mixed material.

Cont'd Directions ▶

6. Rinse and dry area where restoration is to be placed and then place material into prepared tooth structure.

7. Contour material to the proper shape with plastic instrument, if needed, and use a Mylar Matrix Band to hold material in the proper shape while it sets.

8. Complete initial finishing of the material with a finishing bur and paint a protective sealant such as varnish on the outer surface of the restoration.

9. Complete final polishing of restoration 24 hours later.

Special Notes/Helpful Hints • Glass ionomer restorations are "tooth-colored" but opaque in appearance and their esthetics are inferior to dental composites. • Glass ionomer chemically bonds to enamel and dentin and releases fluoride over time. The fluoride released by the material decreases over time but can be recharged with topical fluoride application. • Placement of chemical-cured glass ionomer restorations is technique sensitive. Mixing too slowly or delaying placement of the mixed material causes the adhesive property of the material to be lost. • Glass ionomer materials are susceptible to dehydration, which causes surface crazing. • It takes 24 hours for a glass ionomer restoration to set fully.

■ MATERIAL Glass Ionomer Restorative Materials (Chemically Activated): Single-Dose Capsules

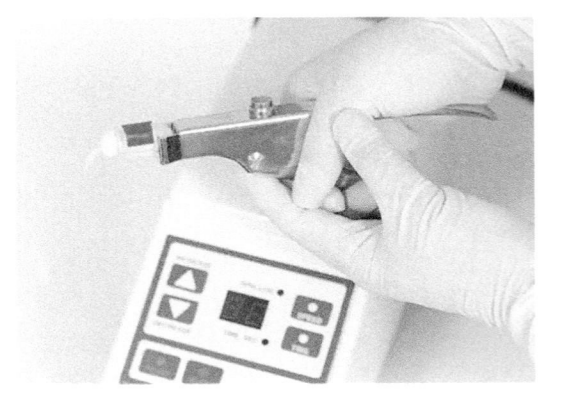

How Supplied ▶ Powder and liquid or single-dose capsules

Composition ▶ Powder—aluminosilicate glass
Liquid—polymers and copolymers of acrylic acid

• Glass ionomer restorative material • Dispensing gun
• Amalgamator • Restorative instruments

Directions ▶ For single-dose capsule systems:

1. Activate capsule, if indicated by manufacturer.
2. Triturate capsule for amount of time indicated by manufacturer.
3. Rinse and dry area where restoration is to be placed and then place material into prepared tooth structure.
4. Contour material to the proper shape with a plastic instrument; if needed, use a Mylar Matrix Band to hold material in the proper shape while it sets.
5. Complete initial finishing of the material with a finishing bur and paint a protective sealant such as varnish on the outer surface of restoration.
6. Complete final polishing of restoration 24 hours later.

▶ Special Notes/Helpful Hints • Glass ionomer restorations are "tooth-colored" but opaque in appearance, which causes their esthetics to be inferior to dental composites. • Glass ionomer chemically bonds to enamel and dentin and releases fluoride over time. The fluoride released by the material decreases over time but can be recharged with topical fluoride application. • Placement of chemical-cured glass ionomer restorations is technique sensitive. Mixing too slowly or delaying placement of the mixed material causes the adhesive property of the material to be lost. • Glass ionomer materials are susceptible to dehydration, which causes surface crazing. • It takes 24 hours for a glass ionomer restoration to set fully.

■ **MATERIAL** Compomers

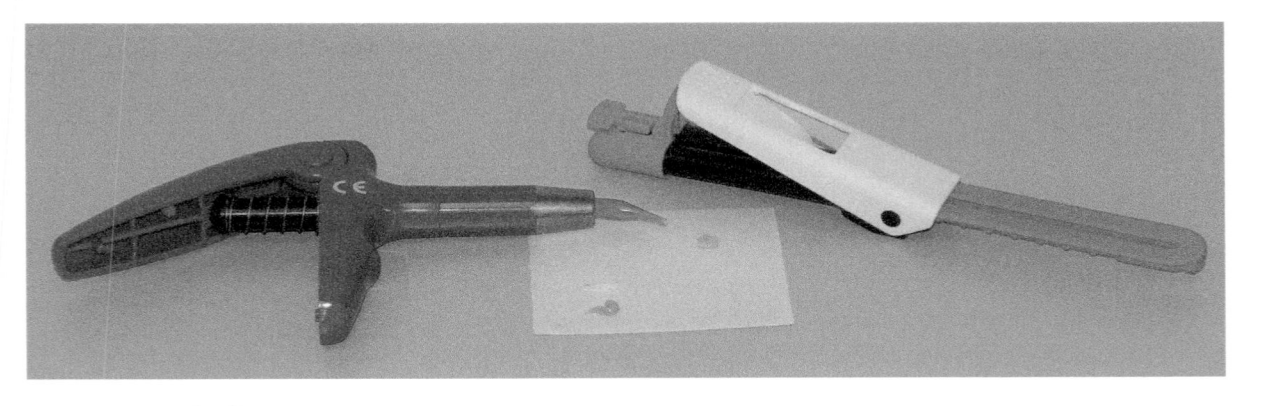

How Supplied ▶ Prepackaged single use cartridges
As a catalyst and base that must be dispensed, mixed, and loaded into a single use cartridge

Composition ▶ Monomer and silicate glass

Armamentarium ▶
- Compomer
- Composite gun
- Etchant
- Bonding system

- Curing light
- Restorative instruments
- Composite placement instrument

Directions ▶
1. Etch tooth surface with 37% orthophosphoric acid.
2. Rinse lightly and dry.
3. Prepare etched tooth surface with primer and bonding agent.
4. Place compomer material in desired location and shape with plastic instrument. If needed, use a Mylar Matrix Band to hold material in the proper shape while it sets.
5. Polymerize with curing light.
6. Adjust and finish material.

◀▶ Special Notes/Helpful Hints • Compomers are a combination of glass ionomer materials and composite and dentin bonding systems. The material initially releases some fluoride, but clinical data showing a reduction in recurrent caries are lacking. This material is recommended for patients with medium risk of caries. • Material is handled similar to composites. • Few compomers are currently available on the market because of the advances in composites. • In contrast to resin-modified glass ionomer, this material requires the use of bonding due to the resin content in the material.

Provisional Restorative Materials

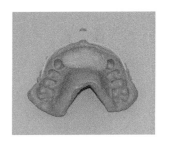

■ MATERIAL Customized Provisional (Bis-Acryl)

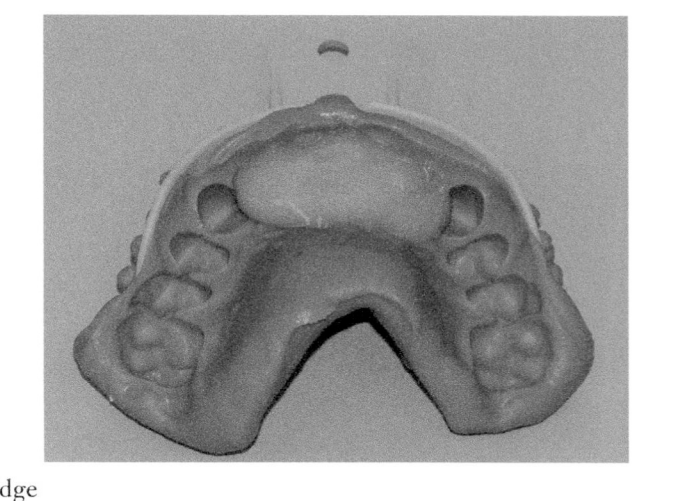

How Supplied ▶ Cartridge

Composition ▶ Dimethacrylate polymer

- Restorative instruments
- Impression material
- Impression tray
- Dispensing gun
- Acrylic cartridge with mixing tip
- High-speed handpiece
- Finishing bur
- Low-speed handpiece
- Round bur
- Temporary cement

Directions ▶

1. Take impression of tooth being restored before tooth is prepared. Impression material used depends on how long the tooth will be in a temporary provisional.
   - Alginate can be used to impress for a temporary intended to be worn for a short time.
   - Another impression material, such as putty, can be used if the temporary will be worn for a longer time. The putty impression can be stored for a longer period without distortion in case the temporary needs to be remade.

Cont'd Directions ▶

2. For a second time, try in the impression to ensure the impression seats properly prior to dispensing acrylic material.

3. Dispense a small amount of acrylic on tray or gauze square, and then continue to dispense acrylic material into the portion of the impression where the tooth was prepared. Ensure tooth is filled to the brim or the margin of the prepared tooth.

4. Reseat impression intraorally with acrylic material in it. Allow impression to remain seated until the small bit of material on tray or gauze square is set.

5. Remove impression from mouth and remove provisional from impression.

6. Reseat provisional on prepared tooth to check fit.

7. Remove flash from margin of provisional and reset to ensure provisional covers prepared tooth and interproximal contact areas are sufficient.

8. Check occlusion with articulating paper and adjust any areas where provisional is too high.

9. Fill provisional with temporary cement and reset on prepared tooth.

10. Remove excess cement after temporary cement has set.

• A custom provisional is also known as a temporary provisional. • A temporary is intended to be temporary; the material used to make the temporary is not strong enough to remain in the mouth for an extended time.

MATERIAL ■ Heat-Activated Dental Acrylic Resins

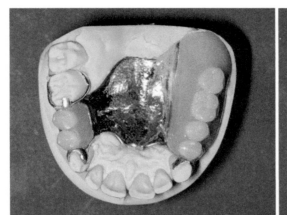
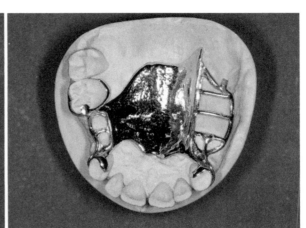

From Hatrick, Eakle, and Bird, 2011.

How Supplied ◀ Powder and liquid

Composition ◀ Acrylic, methyl methacrylate

Armamentarium ▶

- Restorative instruments
- Heat-activated dental acrylic resin
- Mixing bowl
- Mixing spatula
- Hot water bath

Directions ▶ This dental material is used in a dental laboratory setting and arrives to the dental office as a custom order.

1. Mix powder and liquid together to a dough consistency.
2. Mold dough into desired shape.
3. Heat material in temperature-controlled water bath to polymerize material for 8 hours.

▶ Special Notes/Helpful Hints • Most complete and partial dentures use heat-activated acrylic resins for the denture base. The denture base is the pink plastic part of a denture that simulates the gingiva and the lost alveolar bone. • Addition polymerization is an exothermic reaction, and the increase in temperature can become dangerous if the material is left intraorally for extended periods.

■ MATERIAL Chemically-Activated Dental Acrylic Resins

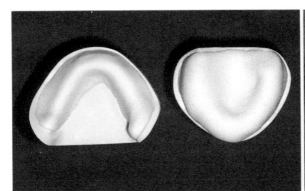 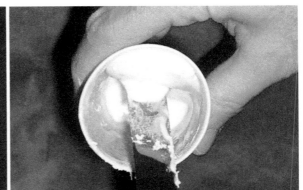

From Hatrick, Eakle, and Bird, 2011.

How Supplied ► Powder and liquid

Composition ► Acrylic and methyl methacrylate

• Maxillary or mandibular edentulous cast
• Chemically-activated dental acrylic resin
• Wax paper cup
• Baseplate wax
• Laboratory handpiece and acrylic bur
• Mixing spatula
• Cast-separating medium and petroleum jelly
• Alcohol torch or burner
• Laboratory knife

Directions ▶ 1. Coat cast with separating medium.
2. Warm sheet of baseplate wax over alcohol torch or burner, and place wax on cast.
3. Adapt wax to cast over edentulous ridges and vestibules using a laboratory knife to trim excess wax.
4. Cut three 2 mm × 2 mm square holes in the wax over the ridges—two in the molar area and one in the incisor area.
5. Mix acrylic powder and liquid together in wax cup in proportions recommended by manufacturer.

◄ Cont'd Directions

6. Apply petroleum jelly to gloved hands.
7. When acrylic mix becomes doughy, form material into a thick rope that is long enough to cover the entire ridge.
8. Adapt resin over wax, into square holes, and into vestibule. Ensure the tray is 1 to 2 mm thick.
9. Cut away excess acrylic material with laboratory knife and mold it into the shape of a handle. Wet the end of the handle that attaches to impression tray with liquid (monomer) and place on tray. Ensure handle is angled in the direction of opposite arch when the tray will be inserted in the mouth to prevent the handle from getting in the way of the lip.
10. Readapt tray material to cast continually while material sets up.
11. After material has cooled, trim edges of tray with acrylic bur to remove excess material and smooth. Final smoothing can be accomplished with flour of pumice and a rag wheel on the dental lathe.
12. Disinfect custom impression tray before use.

Special Notes/Helpful Hints • Chemically-activated dental acrylic resins can be used to make temporary crowns, but most frequently are used for custom impression trays and orthodontic retainers. • Additional polymerization is an exothermic reaction, and the increase in temperature can become dangerous if the material is left intraorally for extended periods.

■ MATERIAL Light-Activated Dental Acrylic Resins

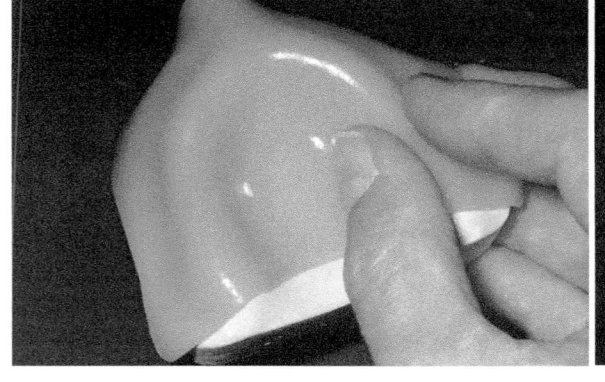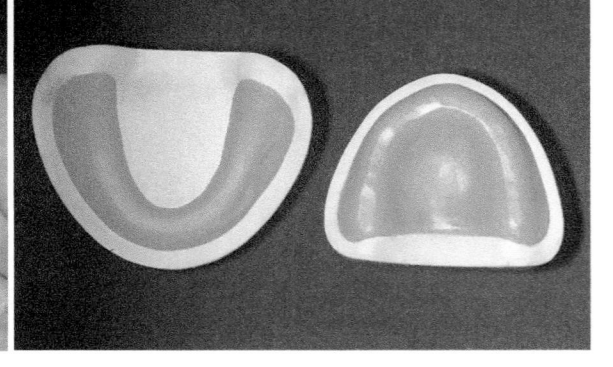

How Supplied ▶ Preformed sheet

Composition ▶ Crystalline silica, polymethyl methacrylate

- Maxillary or mandibular edentulous cast
- Light-activated dental acrylic resin
- Separating medium
- Rubbing alcohol
- Laboratory handpiece and acrylic bur
- Laboratory knife
- Curing light or light-curing unit from manufacturer of product
- Dental lathe and rag wheel
- Pumice

Directions ▶
1. Apply model-separating medium to surface of edentulous cast and allow to dry.
2. Remove sheet of acrylic from protective packaging and place over cast.
3. Press material gently onto cast, ensuring no air is trapped between material and cast.
4. Using a flat blunt instrument, press material into vestibule.
5. Trim away excess material with laboratory knife and smooth edges with fingers.

◄ Cont'd Directions

6. Cut 2-cm-long slit in the back of material in palatal area to allow for shrinkage of material when it is polymerized.

7. Cure material with curing light, or place cast and material into light-curing unit from manufacturer of product. Material should be cured according to manufacturer's instructions.

8. Before final cure of material, place small amount of material over slit that was cut into the palate and cure.

9. After polymerization of material, clean material with rubbing alcohol to remove any film that may be present.

10. Using laboratory handpiece and acrylic bur, trim excess acrylic that extends beyond areas needing to be recorded or to smooth any rough surfaces.

11. Smooth surfaces trimmed with acrylic bur with flour of pumice on a rag wheel using dental lathe.

• Light-activated dental acrylic resin is used to make custom impression trays. • Custom impression trays are used to take final impressions for a full upper or lower denture. • If excess material is present while fabricating the custom tray, it can be used to make a handle on the front of the custom impression tray. • Some manufacturer's may recommend that base plate wax is added to cast prior to the application of the acrylic sheet. The baseplate wax will give additional clearance for the impression material. See directions 2 through 4 under chemically-activated dental acrylic resins.

Intermediate Restorative Material

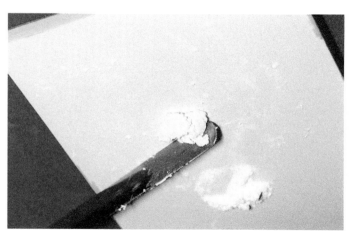

From Hatrick, Eakle, and Bird, 2011.

How Supplied ◄ Powder and liquid

Composition ◄ Zinc oxide, Polymethyl methacrylate, Eugenol, Acetic acid

- Restorative instruments
- Intermediate restorative material
- Mixing pad
- Cement spatula

Directions ▶
1. Isolate tooth where restoration will be placed.
2. Dispense powder and liquid on mixing pad, according to manufacturer's instructions.
3. Incorporate powder into liquid and mix the two together.
4. Roll mixed material into a small ball and place into prepared tooth structure.
5. Use a condenser to pack material into preparation, taking care not to overfill the preparation.
6. Using the blade of a plastic instrument or a Hollenback carver, wipe restorative material toward the margin of the tooth preparation to ensure there is a good seal between the tooth and the restorative material.
7. Use carving instruments to shape the occlusal and to remove any unwanted excess material.

◀▶ Special Notes/Helpful Hints • Some manufacturer's require fluffing of the powder for uniform consistency. • Always recap liquid after dispensing as it will evaporate and may become contaminated if left uncapped. Only dispense liquid on mixing pad immediately prior to mixing material as the liquid will evaporate if left on the mixing pad for an extended period of time. • Material will be stiff during the process of mixing. • Ensure all residual dental materials have been removed from the spatula prior to sterilization. Bacteria can be harbored under the mixed material and live through a sterilization cycle, contributing to cross contamination.

Tooth Whitening

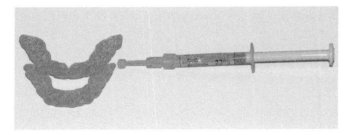

Block-Out Resin

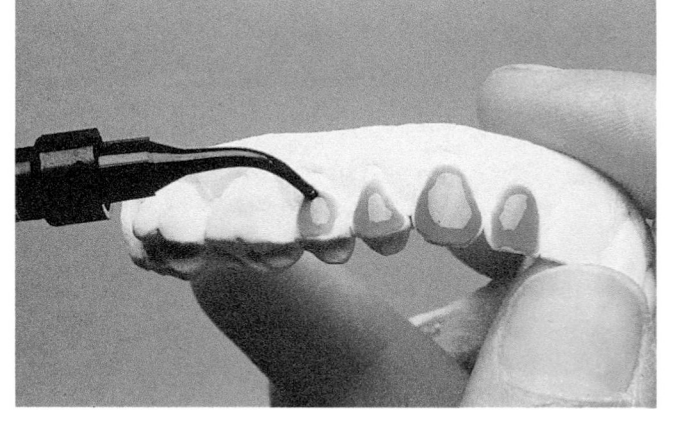

From Hatrick, Eakle, and Bird, 2011.

How Supplied ▶ Liquid in syringe

Composition ▶ Diurethane dimethacrylate
Triethylene glycol dimethacrylate

Armamentarium ▶ • Block-out resin material
• Model
• Curing light
• Shepard's hook explorer

Directions ▶ 1. Extrude block-out resin material onto facial and buccal surfaces of teeth to be whitened, ensuring material is evenly distributed.
2. Smooth any rough areas with explorer or another instrument of choice.
3. Using a curing light, polymerize material for time indicated in manufacturer's instructions.

◀▶ Special Notes/Helpful Hints • Block-out resin is used to form a space between the whitening tray and the tooth structure. This space allows room for whitening gel to sit against the tooth in the whitening tray. • Block-out resin is not a mandatory step in the fabrication of a whitening tray; rather it is a personal preference.

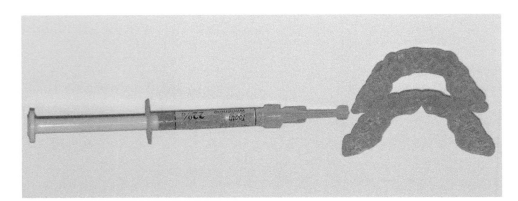

MATERIAL   Hydrogen Peroxide Home Whitening Agent: Tray

How Supplied ◄ Gel in syringe

Composition ◄ Hydrogen peroxide
Glycerin

Armamentarium ▶
- Custom whitening (bleaching) tray
- Whitening gel
- Soft toothbrush
- Paper towel

Directions ▶
1. Brush teeth before inserting trays.
2. Place pea-size amount of whitening gel on the inside of each custom whitening tray toward facial and buccal aspect of each tooth being bleached.
3. Insert trays over teeth and lightly tap to adapt trays to sides of teeth.
4. Use dry or damp paper towel to remove excess material that may have extruded out of trays.

Cont'd Directions ▶

5. Wear trays for time indicated by dentist or manufacturer's instructions.
6. Remove trays from mouth and remove excess gel with soft toothbrush.
7. Rinse twice with water to remove any remaining gel, being sure to expectorate the water; do not swallow.
8. At conclusion of whitening, clean trays with soft brush and cool tap water.
9. Store trays in case provided by dental professional.

Special Notes/Helpful Hints • Whitening products are supplied in different strengths. The strength of the whitening product determines the length of time the product can be worn without causing sensitivity. • Remove excess gel from gingival tissues because peroxide may burn the tissue and cause sloughing if left on the tissue for an extended period. • Hydrogen peroxide is a strong oxidizing agent. People experience more sensitivity with whitening products containing hydrogen peroxide. If a patient experiences sensitivity associated with whitening, he or she should discontinue use of the product and consult a dental professional. • Some whitening products contain fluoride in addition to the standard composition. • Hydrogen peroxide whitening agents are frequently used as in-office professionally-applied systems. • In-office professionally-applied systems are often referred to as power whitening, and the material is activated by light or heat in the form of an ultraviolet light or laser.

■ MATERIAL Carbamide Peroxide Home Whitening Agents: Tray

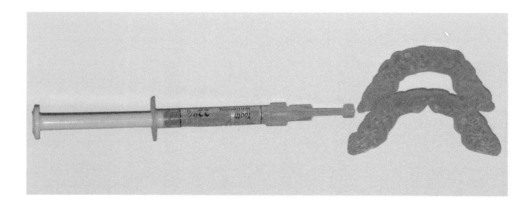

How Supplied ◄ Gel in syringe

Composition ◄ Carbamide peroxide
Glycerin

Armamentarium ▶
- Custom whitening (bleaching) tray
- Whitening gel
- Soft toothbrush
- Paper towel

Directions ▶
1. Brush teeth before inserting trays.
2. Place pea-size amount of whitening gel on the inside of each custom whitening tray toward facial and buccal aspect of each tooth being bleached.
3. Insert trays over teeth and lightly tap to adapt trays to sides of teeth.
4. Use dry or damp paper towel to remove excess material that may have extruded out of trays.
5. Wear trays for time indicated by dentist or manufacturer's instructions.
6. Remove trays from mouth and remove excess gel with soft toothbrush.
7. Rinse twice with water to remove any remaining gel, being sure to expectorate the water; do not swallow.
8. At conclusion of whitening, clean trays with soft brush and cool tap water.
9. Store trays in case provided by dental professional.

▶ Special Notes/Helpful Hints • Whitening products are supplied in different strengths. The strength of the whitening product determines the length of time product can be worn without causing sensitivity. • Remove excess gel from gingival tissues because peroxide may burn the tissue and cause sloughing if left on the tissue for an extended period. • Carbamide peroxide is a weak oxidizing agent. People have a tendency to have less sensitivity associated with carbamide peroxide whitening agents. If a patient experiences sensitivity associated with whitening, he or she should discontinue use of the product and consult a dental professional. • Some whitening products contain fluoride in addition to the standard composition.

MATERIAL ■ Sodium Perborate

Courtesy Sultan Healthcare, Hackensack, NJ.

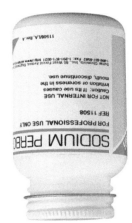

SODIUM PERBO
FOR PROFESSIONAL USE ONLY
REF 11508
NOT FOR INTERNAL USE
Caution: If its use causes
irritation or soreness in the
mouth, discontinue use.
Sultan Chemists, Inc., 85 West Forest Avenue, Englewood
1-800-637-8582 Fax: 1-201-871-0321 http://www.sultanhealthcare
11508LA, Rev. A

How Supplied ◀ Powder

Composition ◀ Sodium perborate

Armamentarium ▶
- Restorative instruments
- Cotton pellets
- Zinc phosphate or intermediate restorative material (IRM)
- Sodium perborate powder
- Dappen dish

Directions ▶
1. Complete endodontic treatment before whitening procedure.
2. Open canal, and remove gutta percha.
3. Mix sodium perborate with water in Dappen dish to make a slurry consistency. Place slurry in open canal and cover with cotton pellets.
4. Seal open canal with zinc phosphate or IRM.
5. Leave whitening solution in tooth structure for 3 to 7 days.
6. Reevaluate patient during time whitening gel is left in the tooth to determine results of whitening.

▶ Special Notes/Helpful Hints • Sodium perborate is a weak oxidizing agent. • This whitening method is considered a walking bleach method because the material is left in the tooth structure for several days. • The bond of esthetic materials can be inhibited by the walking bleach method. Final esthetic restorations on a tooth that has had the walking bleach method completed should be delayed by a minimum of 7 days. • Walking bleach can also cause root resorption. • Because of its side effects, the walking bleach method is not used frequently.

■ **MATERIAL**

In-Office Professionally-Applied Whitening

From Hatrick, Eakle, and Bird, 2011.

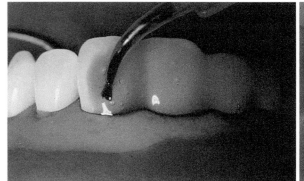
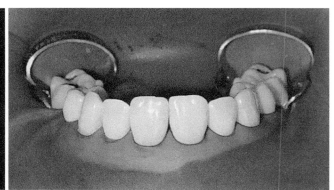

How Supplied ◄ Gel in syringe

Composition ◄ Hydrogen peroxide
Glycerin

• Tinted safety glasses or light shield
• Timing device
• Mouth mirror and explorer
• Slow-speed handpiece and contra-angle
• Pumice
• Gauze
• Dental dam (traditional or liquid)

1. Polish teeth with pumice to remove any soft debris on tooth structure.
2. Record starting shade and take "before" photographs.
3. Place tissue protection on gingiva, lips, and face.
4. Place dental dam isolation, ensuring all tissue is covered.
   • Traditional dental dam
   • Liquid dam

Cont'd Directions ▶ 5. Place bleach on tooth surface, and follow manufacturer's instructions for time and light or heat source application.

6. Suction bleach off of tooth surface with high-volume evacuator and wipe remaining material off with gauze.

7. Repeat steps 5 and 6 until desired shade has been achieved. Manufacturer may recommend a specific limit to application of material to prevent excessive sensitivity.

▶ **Special Notes/Helpful Hints** • Prescription-strength fluoride is recommended for 2 weeks before application of in-office whitening to reduce sensitivity. • In-office application of whitening solution may not be performed by dental auxiliaries in some states. • Additional appointments may be needed to achieve desired shade, or home whitening may be used in conjunction with in-office whitening.

Dental Cements

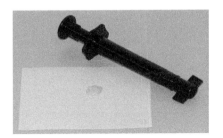

MATERIAL Zinc Oxide–Eugenol Cement (TempBond): Pastes

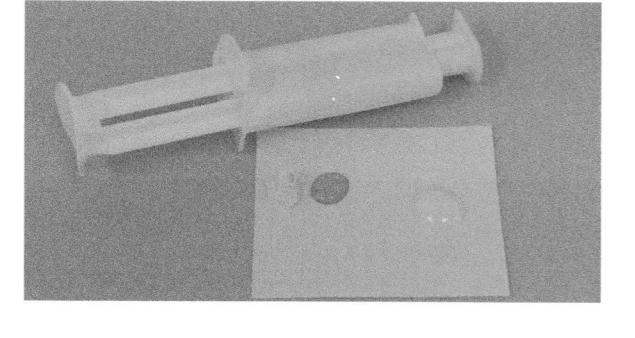

How Supplied ▶ Pastes or powder and liquids

Composition ▶ Zinc oxide, rosin, zinc acetate, and eugenol or mixture of eugenol and other oils

Armamentarium ▶
- Zinc oxide–eugenol cement
- Mixing pad for pastes
- Cement spatula
- Restorative instruments

Directions ▶ For paste systems:

1. Dispense two pastes in equal lengths on a paper mixing pad.
2. Using cement spatula, swirl and whip together pastes vigorously until a homogeneous paste is obtained.
3. Use the side of the spatula to scrape up mixed material and load restoration.
4. Dry area where restoration is to be placed, and then place loaded restoration intraorally.
5. Instruct patient to bite on a gauze square until material is no longer soft or stringy.
6. Clean excess cement from around margin of restoration.

◀▶ Special Notes/Helpful Hints • Most paste systems are used as temporary cements because of their lack of strength and solubility. • Powder and liquid systems are reinforced and can be used for temporary restorations and intermediate bases. • When using the material as a base, the consistency is similar to pie dough. If too little powder is used, the mixture becomes sticky or tacky. A proper base mix does not stick to instruments, allowing for the material to be condensed into a tooth preparation.

MATERIAL

Zinc Oxide–Eugenol Cement (TempBond): Powder and Liquids

How Supplied ▶ Pastes or powder and liquids

Composition ▶ Powder—zinc oxide, rosin, and zinc acetate

Liquid—eugenol or mixture of eugenol and other oils

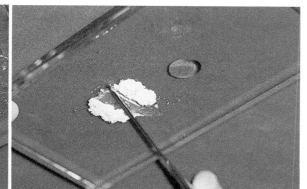

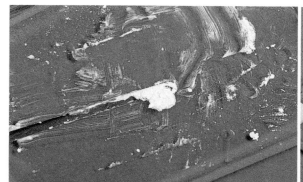

From Hatrick, Eakle, and Bird, 2011.

- Zinc oxide–eugenol cement
- Glass slab for powder and liquid
- Cement spatula
- Restorative instruments

Directions ▶ For powder and liquid systems:

1. Fluff powder by shaking bottle gently.
2. Measure powder using scoop provided by manufacturer, and dispense onto glass slab.
3. Dispense liquid as droplets onto glass slab.
4. Force powder into liquid, using large increments of powder followed by smaller increments.
5. For cementation, the consistency results in material that can be pulled up into a "1 inch" string when the flat surface of cement spatula is pulled from mixed material.
6. Use the side of the spatula to scrape up mixed material and load restoration.
7. Dry area where restoration is to be placed, and then place loaded restoration intraorally.
8. Instruct patient to bite on a gauze square until material has set and becomes rigid.
9. Clean excess material from around margin of restoration.

◀▶ Special Notes/Helpful Hints • Most paste systems are used as temporary cements because of their lack of strength and solubility. • Powder and liquid systems are reinforced and can be used for temporary restorations and intermediate bases. • When using the material as a base, the consistency is similar to pie dough. If too little powder is used, the mixture becomes sticky or tacky. A proper base mix does not stick to instruments, allowing for the material to be condensed into a tooth preparation.

■ MATERIAL   Zinc Phosphate Cement

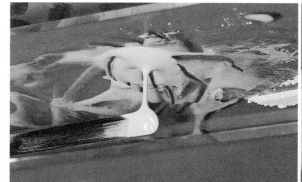
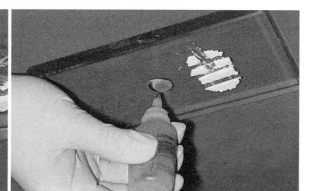

From Hatrick, Eakle, and Bird, 2011.

How Supplied ◄ Powder and liquid

Composition ◄ Powder—zinc oxide, magnesium oxide, and pigments
Liquid—phosphoric acid in water

• Zinc phosphate cement
• Chilled glass slab
• Broad cement spatula
• Restorative instruments

1. Fluff powder by shaking bottle gently.
2. Measure powder using scoop provided by manufacturer, and dispense onto chilled glass slab.
3. Divide powder into four to six small mounds or increments.
4. Dispense liquid as droplets onto chilled glass slab.
5. Force one increment of powder into liquid and slowly mix for 10 to 15 seconds.
6. Force second increment of powder into liquid and slowly mix for 10 to 15 seconds. Continue to add powder to the mixture in small increments until proper consistency has been reached.
7. For cementation, the consistency results in material that can be pulled up into a "1 inch" string when the flat surface of cement spatula is pulled from mixed material.

▶ **Cont'd Directions**

8. Use the side of the spatula to scrape up mixed material and load restoration.
9. Dry area where restoration is to be placed, and then place loaded restoration intraorally.
10. Instruct patient to bite on a gauze square until material has set and becomes rigid.
11. Clean excess material from around margin of restoration.

If the material is being used for a base, the consistency will allow for the material to be rolled into a ball. If too little powder is used, the mixture is sticky or tacky. Before placing the base, the ball should be rolled in cement powder to prevent the material from sticking to instruments during placement. A proper base mix does not stick to instruments if the ball of material and instruments are covered with cement powder.

Special Notes/Helpful Hints • A chilled glass slab is essential with use of this material because of the exothermic reaction that occurs during mixing. If the material is mixed over a larger surface area of the chilled glass slab, the slab absorbs the heat from the exothermic reaction. • The material has a low pH until it has set, which causes the material to be irritating to the pulp. Because of the low pH, a varnish is often placed when this material is intended to be used as a base.

■ **MATERIAL** Zinc Polycarboxylate Cement

How Supplied ◄ Powder and liquid

Composition ◄ Powder—zinc oxide
Liquid—polyacrylic acid in water

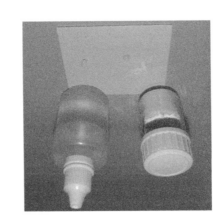

• Polycarboxylate cement
• Wax-coated disposable mixing pad
• Cement spatula
• Restorative instruments

Directions ▶ 1. Shake bottle of powder gently.
2. Measure powder using scoop provided by manufacturer, and dispense onto mixing pad.
3. Dispense liquid as droplets onto mixing pad.
4. Force about 90% of powder into liquid and mix quickly to ensure a mixing time of 30 to 60 seconds is not exceeded. The remaining powder is added to adjust consistency.
5. Use the side of the spatula to scrape up mixed material and load restoration.
6. Dry area where restoration is to be placed, and then place loaded restoration intraorally.
7. Instruct patient to bite on gauze square until material has set and becomes rigid.
8. Clean excess material from around the margin of restoration.

▶ Special Notes/Helpful Hints • Zinc polycarboxylate cement is not very strong and has moderate solubility. • The proper consistency of the material appears creamy. • The cement is no longer usable when it loses its luster or becomes stringy. • Working time for cement is about 3 minutes after mixing. • A chilled glass slab can be used to allow for a longer working time.

■ MATERIAL Glass Ionomer Cement: Powder and Liquid

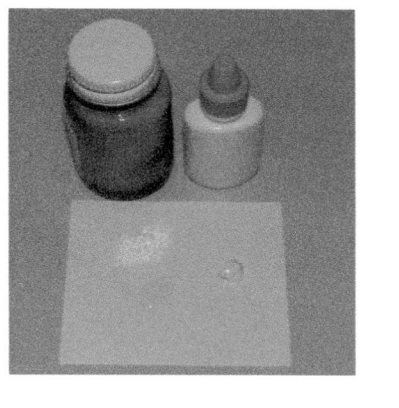

How Supplied ▶ Powder and liquid
Premeasured single-dose capsule

Composition ▶ Powder—finely ground aluminosilicate glass
Liquid—polycarboxylate copolymer in water

• Glass ionomer cement
• Wax-coated mixing pad

• Cement spatula
• Restorative instruments

Directions ▶ For powder and liquid systems:

1. Tumble bottle of powder gently.
2. Measure powder using scoop provided by manufacturer, and dispense onto mixing pad.
3. Dispense liquid as droplets onto mixing pad.
4. Divide powder into two equal portions.
5. Force first half of powder into liquid with stiff spatula and then add second portion. Mix quickly to ensure a mixing time of 30 to 60 seconds is not exceeded.
6. Use the side of the spatula to scrape up mixed material and load restoration.
7. Dry area where restoration is to be placed, and then place loaded restoration intraorally.
8. Instruct patient to bite on gauze square until material has set and becomes rigid.
9. Clean excess material from around margin of restoration.

◀▶ Special Notes/Helpful Hints • Manufacturer's recommended powder-to-liquid ratios should be followed. • A cooled mixing slab slows the setting reaction and provides additional working time. • Glass ionomer should not be used when it is no longer glossy. • During application, contact with water should be avoided and the field should be isolated. • Cement sets in the mouth in about 7 minutes from the start of mixing. • Glass ionomer releases fluoride, which allows material to have an anticariogenic effect.

MATERIAL Glass Ionomer Cement: Premeasured Single-Dose Capsule

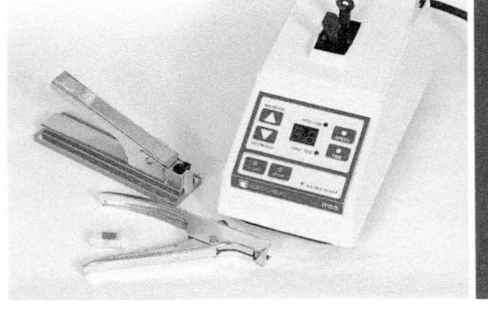
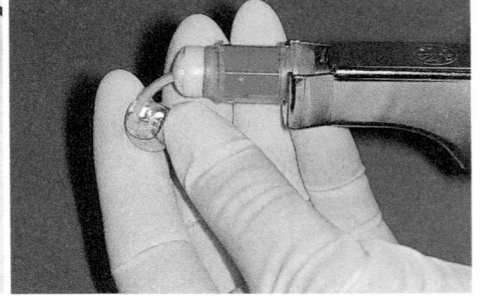

How Supplied ▶ Powder and liquid or pastes
Premeasured single-dose capsule

Composition ▶ Powder—finely ground aluminosilicate glass
Liquid—polycarboxylate copolymer in water

Armamentarium ▶
- Glass ionomer cement capsule
- Capsule activator (if indicated)
- Dispensing gun
- Cement spatula
- Restorative instruments
- Triturator

Directions ▶ For single-dose capsule systems:

1. Activate capsule, if indicated by manufacturer.
2. Triturate capsule for amount of time indicated by manufacturer.
3. Load capsule into dispensing syringe provided by manufacturer and dispense material into restoration.
4. Dry area where restoration is to be placed, and then place loaded restoration intraorally.
5. Instruct patient to bite on gauze square until material has set and becomes rigid.
6. Clean excess material from around margin of restoration.

◀▶ Special Notes/Helpful Hints • Manufacturer's recommended powder-to-liquid ratios should be followed. • A cooled glass mixing slab slows the setting reaction and provides additional working time. • Glass ionomer should not be used when it is no longer glossy. • During application, contact with water should be avoided, and the field should be isolated. • The cement sets in the mouth in about 7 minutes from the start of mixing. • Glass ionomer releases fluoride, which allows material to have an anticariogenic effect.

■ **MATERIAL**

Resin-Modified Glass Ionomer Cement:
Powder and Liquid

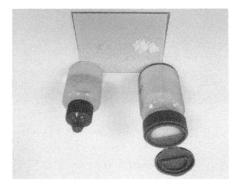

◀ **How Supplied** Powder and liquid or pastes

Premeasured single-dose capsule

◀ **Composition** Powder—radiopaque aluminosilicate glass

Liquid—monomers, polyacrylic acid, and water

Armamentarium ▶
- Resin-modified glass ionomer cement
- Wax-coated mixing pad
- Cement spatula
- Restorative instruments

Directions ▶ For powder and liquid systems:

1. Tumble bottle of powder gently.
2. Measure powder using scoop provided by manufacturer, and dispense onto mixing pad.
3. Holding bottle vertically, dispense liquid as droplets onto mixing pad.
4. Quickly force powder into liquid with stiff spatula to ensure a mixing time of 30 seconds is not exceeded. Material should have a mousselike consistency.
5. Use the side of the spatula to scrape up mixed material and load restoration.
6. Dry area where restoration is to be placed, and then place loaded restoration intraorally.
7. Instruct patient to bite on gauze square until material has set and becomes rigid.
8. Clean excess material from around margin of restoration.

◀▶ Special Notes/Helpful Hints • The working time of resin-modified glass ionomer cement is 2.5 minutes. • Cement is applied to a clean, dry tooth that is not desiccated.

MATERIAL Resin-Modified Glass Ionomer Cement: Premeasured Single-Dose Capsule

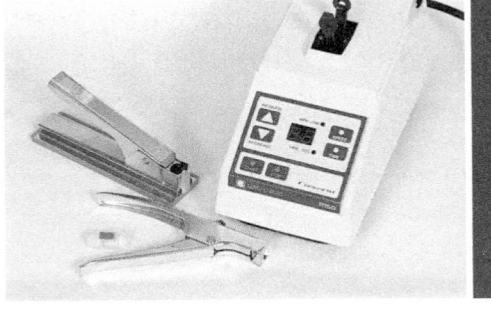 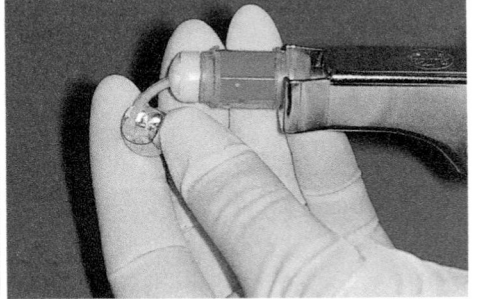

How Supplied ▶ Powder and liquid or pastes
Premeasured single-dose capsule

Composition ▶ Powder—radiopaque aluminosilicate glass
Liquid—monomers, polyacrylic acid, and water

• Resin-modified glass ionomer cement capsule
- Capsule activator (if indicated)
- Dispensing syringe
- Cement spatula
- Restorative instruments
- Triturator

Directions ▶ For single-dose capsule systems:

1. Activate capsule, if indicated by manufacturer.
2. Triturate capsule for amount of time indicated by manufacturer.
3. Load capsule into dispensing syringe provided by manufacturer and dispense material into restoration.
4. Dry area where restoration is to be placed, and then place loaded restoration intraorally.
5. Instruct patient to bite on gauze square until material has set and becomes rigid.
6. Clean excess material from around margin of restoration.

◀▶ Special Notes/Helpful Hints • Working time of resin-modified glass ionomer cement is 2.5 minutes. • Cement is applied to a clean, dry tooth that is not desiccated.

MATERIAL Esthetic Resin Cement: Two Pastes

How Supplied ▶ Single paste (light-activated)
Two pastes (dual-cure)

Composition ▶ Dimethacrylate resin and glass filler

• Etchant
  • Orthophosphoric acid gel
  • Hydrofluoric acid gel
- Dual-cure dentinal bonding agent
- Esthetic resin cement
- Wax-coated mixing pad (needed for two-paste system)
- Plastic cement spatula (needed for two-paste system)
- Restorative instruments

Directions ▶ For preparation of restoration:

1. Prepare restoration by coating inside of restoration with hydrofluoric acid for period of time indicated by manufacturer.
2. Rinse etchant from restoration, and dry with compressed air.
3. Paint silane agent on etched interior portion of restoration.

◄ Cont'd Directions

For preparation of tooth structure:

1. Prepare tooth structure by coating prepared surface with 37% orthophosphoric acid.
2. Rinse etchant and dry with compressed air.
3. Keep area isolated to ensure no contamination from debris or saliva occurs.
4. Paint tooth structure with bonding agent, and light cure according to manufacturer's instructions.
5. Mix equal amounts of esthetic resin cement on wax mixing pad with plastic cement spatula.
6. Scrape up material with cement spatula and load into prepared restoration.
7. Ensure tooth structure has been isolated and no contamination has occurred and place restoration on tooth structure.
8. Cure according to manufacturer's instructions.

▶ Special Notes/Helpful Hints • Follow manufacturer's recommendations for etching, rinsing, drying, and curing times. • Composite cements come in various shades and can change the appearance of an esthetic restoration. • These cements are used for bonding all-ceramic and indirect composite restorations. • Esthetic, adhesive, and self-adhesive types of resin cements are available. The different types may require fewer or more steps when manipulating.

■ MATERIAL Esthetic Resin Cement: Single Paste

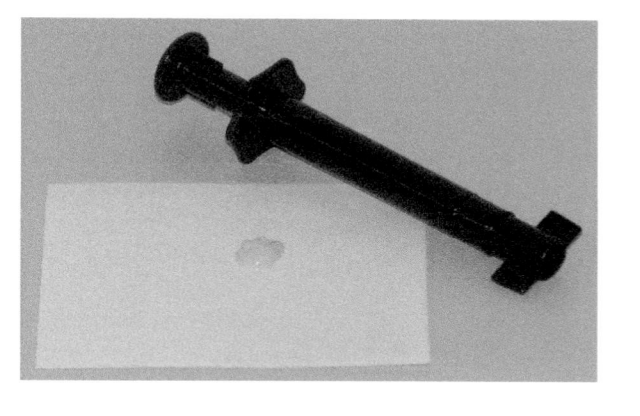

How Supplied ▶ Single paste (light-activated)

Two pastes (dual-cure)

Composition ▶ Dimethacrylate resin and glass filler

• Etchant
  • Orthophosphoric acid gel
  • Hydrofluoric acid gel
• Dual-cure dentinal bonding agent
• Esthetic resin cement
• Restorative instruments

Directions ▶ For preparation of restoration:

1. Prepare restoration by coating inside of restoration with hydrofluoric acid for period of time indicated by manufacturer.
2. Rinse etchant from restoration, and dry with compressed air.
3. Paint silane agent on etched interior portion of restoration.

Cont'd Directions ◄

For preparation of tooth structure:

1. Prepare tooth structure by coating prepared surface with 37% orthophosphoric acid.
2. Rinse etchant and dry with compressed air.
3. Keep area isolated to ensure no contamination from debris or saliva occurs.
4. Paint tooth structure with bonding agent and light cure according to manufacturer's instructions.
5. Dispense composite cement into prepared restoration and place on prepared tooth structure.
6. Polymerize composite cement with curing light, according to manufacturer's instructions.

Special Notes/Helpful Hints • Follow manufacturer's recommendations for etching, rinsing, drying, and curing times. • Composite cements come in various shades and can change the appearance of an esthetic restoration. • These cements are used for bonding all-ceramic and indirect composite restorations. • Esthetic, adhesive, and self-adhesive types of resin cements are available. The different types may require fewer or more steps when manipulating.

Impression Materials: Elastomers, Inelastic or Rigid Impression Materials, and Hydrocolloids

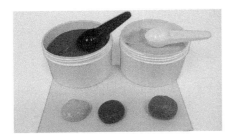

■ **MATERIAL** Polyether (Elastomer)

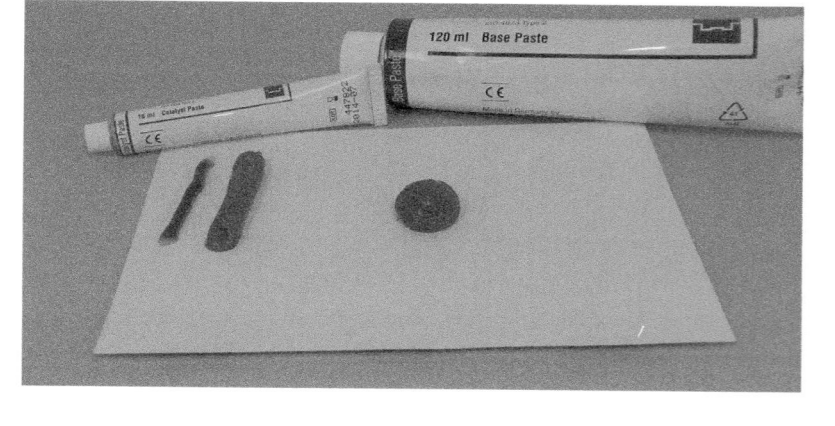

How Supplied ▶ Two pastes in tubes: gray base paste and red accelerator paste

Composition ▶ Base—organic polymer, reinforcing agents
Accelerator—citric ester, silica, polyethylene glycol

Armamentarium ▶
- Polyether impression material
- Mixing spatula
- Wax-coated mixing pad
- Impression tray

Directions ▶
1. Dispense equal lengths of base and catalyst onto wax-coated mixing pad.
2. Mix both pastes together for 45 seconds (homogeneous mix should be obtained).
3. Scoop mixed material onto end of mixing spatula, load into impression tray, and take impression.

◀▮▶ Special Notes/Helpful Hints • When mixing vinyl polyether silicones, do not mix by stirring (to avoid formation of bubbles). Wait a minimum of 30 minutes from the conclusion of taking an impression to pour model. • See manufacturer's instructions for specific processing and setting times.

- **MATERIAL** Addition Silicone: Vinyl Polysiloxane (Elastomer)

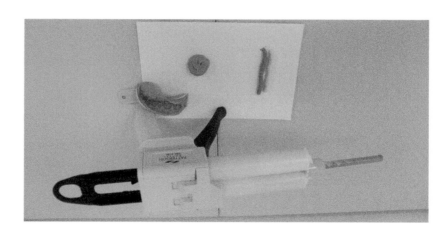

How Supplied ▶ Different-colored pastes in cartridges or containers

Composition ▶ Silicone, reinforcing filler, and chloroplatinic acid

Armamentarium ▶
- Double-bite tray
- Addition silicone impression material in cartridges
- Dispenser gun
- Mixing tips
- Impression syringe
- Paper towel

Directions ▶
1. Isolate quadrant in which impression will be made.
2. Take preassembled dispenser gun and mixing tip and extrude small portion of material on a paper towel; when homogeneous mix is observed, dispense material into impression syringe.
3. Using impression syringe, dispense material around prepared tooth structure.
4. Load double-bite impression tray with impression material and place over prepared tooth structure.
5. Instruct patient to bite together.
6. Allow material to set or harden. Once hardened (this can be verified by touching the small amount extruded onto the paper towel) the impression may be removed.
7. Verify that all components of the prepared tooth have been recorded in the impression and no voids are present.

◀▮▶ Special Notes/Helpful Hints • Addition silicone is available in light, medium, and heavy body. • Light-bodied material is best used for a double-bite impression or the wash of a two-step putty technique.

■ **MATERIAL**

Addition Silicone: Putty Vinyl Polysiloxane (Elastomer)

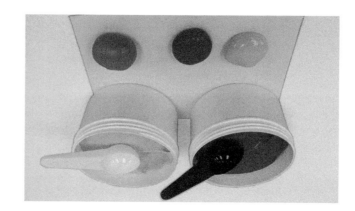

How Supplied ◄ Different-colored pastes in cartridges or containers

Composition ◄ Silicone, reinforcing filler, and chloroplatinic acid

• Double-bite tray or quadrant impression tray
• Elastomeric impression material in containers
• Scoops

Directions ▶ 1. Isolate quadrant in which impression will be made.
2. Take premeasured balls of material and begin kneading materials together with clean bare hands.
3. When homogeneous mix is obtained, place material in impression tray and take impression.

◀▮▷ Special Notes/Helpful Hints • Material comes in light, medium, and heavy body. • Heavy-bodied material such as putty is often used to take an impression of a tooth before preparation for a restoration.

■ MATERIAL Polysulfide (Elastomer)

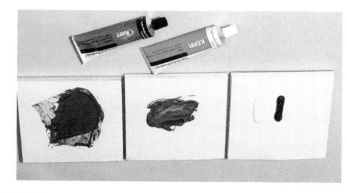

From Hatrick, Eakle, and Bird, 2011.

How Supplied ◄ Two pastes in tubes: white base paste and brown accelerator paste

Composition ◄ Base—organic polymer, reinforcing agents
Accelerator—lead oxide, inert oils

NOTE: Mixing pad in middle or second mixing pad shows material not fully mixed.

Armamentarium ▶ • Polysulfide material
• Mixing pad
• Impression material spatula
• Impression tray

Directions ▶ 1. Dispense two pastes in equal lengths on paper mixing pad.
2. Using an impression material spatula, swirl and whip together pastes vigorously until homogeneous paste is obtained (mixing may take 30 to 90 seconds).
3. Use the side of the spatula blade to scrape up mixed material and load material into impression tray.
4. Place loaded impression tray intraorally to take impression.

Special Notes/Helpful Hints • The polymerization process begins when mixing begins and then proceeds slowly. • This material is more accurate than alginate, but there are other nonaqueous elastomeric materials that are more accurate. • The impression should be poured within several hours after taking the impression. • Custom impression trays are recommended for optimal results.

■ **MATERIAL** Impression Plaster (Inelastic or Rigid Impression Material)

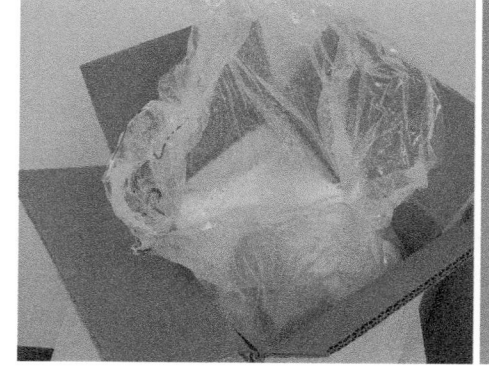
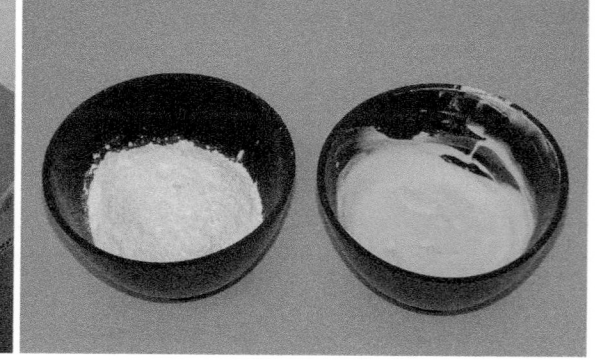

How Supplied ▶ Powder

Composition ▶ Calcium sulfate hemihydrate

- Impression plaster
- Scoop or scale for weighing material if material is supplied in bulk container
- Water measurer with milliliter markings
- Mixing bowl
- Spatula
- Impression trays

Directions ▶

1. Place impression plaster in mixing bowl; if plaster is supplied in a bulk container, measure appropriate amount of plaster needed using a scale, and always use measuring scoop supplied by manufacturer when available.
2. Measure water using calibrated water measurer with milliliter markings.
3. Gently stir together powder and water.
4. Once powder has been wetted by all the water, increase mixing efforts.
5. Place mixing bowl on vibrator to push any air bubbles incorporated in mixture to the surface. Incorporation of air bubbles in the mix distorts impression.
6. Load impression tray with impression plaster and place in patient's mouth.
7. Remove impression tray with a quick motion after material has set.

◀▶ Special Notes/Helpful Hints • Impression plaster differs from other gypsum products because it has flavor added; these plasters set more quickly to minimize the time material is in the mouth. • This material is considered rigid and should be used only to take impressions of an edentulous area of the mouth.

■ **MATERIAL**

Impression Compound (Inelastic or Rigid Impression Material)

How Supplied ◂ Sticks or cakes

Composition ◂ Resins, waxes, organic acids, fillers, and coloring agents

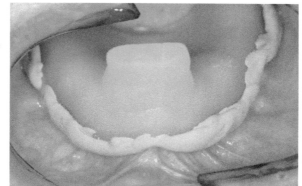

From Hatrick, Eakle, and Bird, 2011; *left*, courtesy Dr. Mark Dellinges.

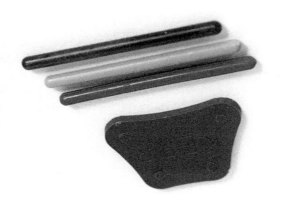

• Impression compound
• Compound heater
• Impression tray

1. Plug compound heater in and turn on.
2. Place water in chamber of compound heater if chamber is empty.
3. Place impression compound in impression tray and place both tray and impression compound in compound heater.
4. When material has softened, place impression tray intraorally to take impression.
5. Remove impression tray from patient's mouth after material has cooled to mouth temperature.
6. A water spray can be used to assist in cooling process.

◀▮▶ Special Notes/Helpful Hints • Impression compound is wax with added filler to improve handling and stability. • This material is often used for preliminary impressions for complete dentures. • Final impressions are taken with a material that is better suited to record fine details.

■ **MATERIAL**

Zinc Oxide–Eugenol Impression Material (Inelastic or Rigid Impression Material)

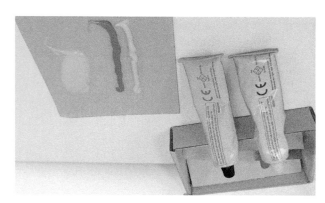

◄ **How Supplied** — Two pastes in tubes: white base paste and red accelerator paste

◄ **Composition** — Base—zinc oxide, olive oil

Accelerator—oil of cloves, rosin, filler particles, lanoline, accelerator solution

Armamentarium ▶
- Zinc oxide–eugenol impression pastes
- Mixing pad
- Impression material spatula
- Impression tray

Directions ▶
1. Dispense two pastes in equal lengths on paper mixing pad.
2. Using impression material spatula, swirl, whip vigorously, and scrape together pastes until homogeneous paste is obtained.
3. Use side of spatula blade to scoop up mixed material, and load material into impression tray.
4. Place loaded impression tray intraorally to take impression.

Special Notes/Helpful Hints • Zinc oxide–eugenol impression material sets to a hard rigid mass, which limits its use to edentulous ridges. • This material is commonly used in custom trays for the final impression for a complete denture. • Initial set of material occurs in 3 to 5 minutes. Final setting time is less than 10 minutes.

■ **MATERIAL** Alginate: Irreversible Hydrocolloid (Hydrocolloid)

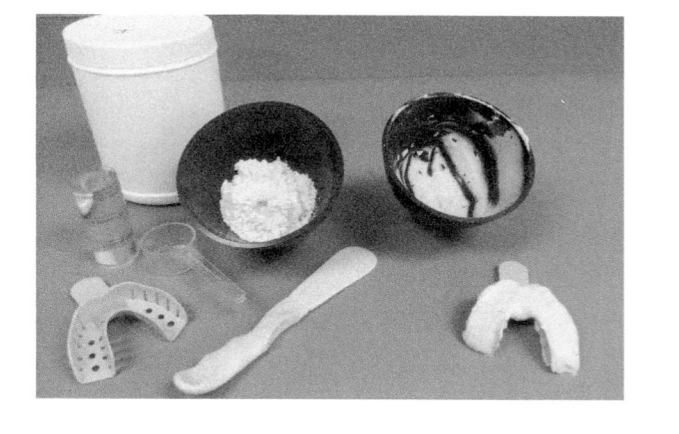

How Supplied ▶ Powder

Composition ▶ Potassium, calcium sulfate dehydrate, potassium sulfate, trisodium phosphate, and diatomaceous earth

- Alginate material
- Scoop if material is supplied in bulk container
- Water measurer
- Mixing bowl
- Spatula
- Impression trays

Directions ►

1. Place alginate in mixing bowl; if alginate is supplied in a bulk container, fluff by shaking container before measuring out, and always use measuring scoop supplied by manufacturer.
2. Measure water using calibrated water measurer also supplied by manufacturer and add water to mixing bowl with alginate.
3. Gently stir together powder and water.
4. Once powder has been wetted by all the water, increase mixing efforts.
5. Push paste against side of mixing bowl to force water and powder together.
6. Continue spatulation until mix is smooth and creamy (typical mixing time is 1 minute).
7. Load impression tray with alginate material and place in patient's mouth.
8. Remove impression tray with a quick motion after material has set.

◀▶ Special Notes/Helpful Hints • Alginate is supplied in regular-set material, which gels in 3 to 4 minutes, and fast-set material, which gels in 1 to 2 minutes. • The setting time of a material can be altered with water temperature. The hotter the water, the faster the material gels. • Water in alginate evaporates quickly, requiring impressions to be poured within 30 minutes after an impression has been taken.

Gypsum Products

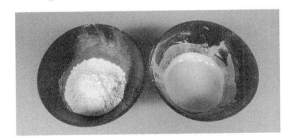

MATERIAL Model Plaster

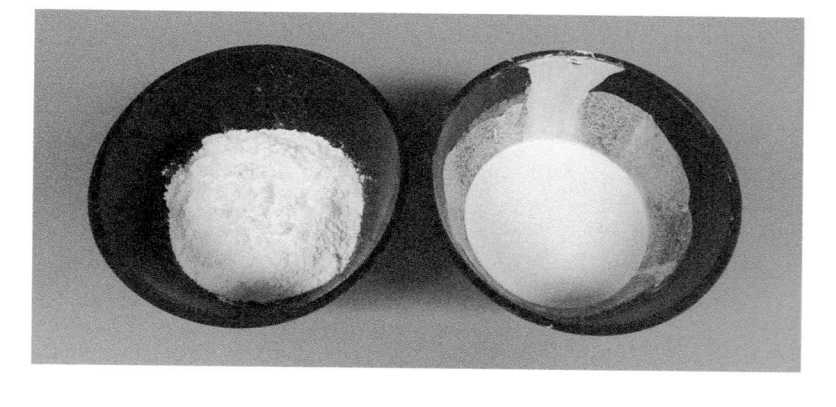

How Supplied ▶ Powder

Composition ▶ Beta-calcium sulfate hemihydrate

Armamentarium ▶
- Plaster
- Two flexible mixing bowls
- Mixing spatula
- Water measurer with milliliter markings
- Dental vibrator
- Balance or scale
- Unpoured impression

Directions ▶
1. Measure 100 g of plaster and place in first mixing bowl.
2. Measure 45 to 50 mL of room temperature water and place in second mixing bowl.
3. Gradually add preweighed powder to water.
4. Combine powder and water by mixing the two together using mixing spatula.
5. Place mixed plaster onto dental vibrator while holding pressure against bowl on dental vibrator.
6. Fill impression using dental vibrator to reduce air bubbles, and allow material to flow into impression.
7. Place filled impression on flat surface away from dental vibrator, and allow to dry.

◀▶ Special Notes/Helpful Hints • Plaster is used when strength is not critical. • Follow specific manufacturer's instructions for recommendations on powder-to-water ratios. • A graduated cylinder can be used for measuring water because 1 g of water has a volume very close to 1 mL. • Preweighed envelops of gypsum products are available to eliminate need for weighing. • Plaster is often white in color; however, manufacturers can add colorants to change color of powder.

■ **MATERIAL**

Dental Stone

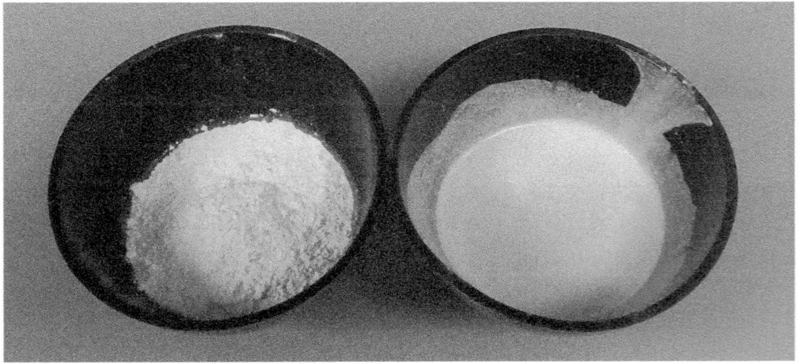

How Supplied ◄ Powder

Composition ◄ Alpha-calcium sulfate hemihydrate

- Stone
- Two flexible mixing bowls
- Mixing spatula
- Water measurer with milliliter markings
- Dental vibrator
- Balance or scale
- Unpoured impression

Directions ▶ 1. Measure 100 g of stone and place in first mixing bowl.
2. Measure 30 to 32 mL of room temperature water and place in second mixing bowl.
3. Gradually add preweighed powder to water.
4. Combine powder and water by mixing the two together using mixing spatula.
5. Place mixed stone onto dental vibrator while holding pressure against bowl on dental vibrator.
6. Fill impression using dental vibrator to reduce air bubbles, and allow material to flow into impression.
7. Place filled impression on flat surface away from dental vibrator, and allow to dry.

◀▶ Special Notes/Helpful Hints • Stone is stronger and more expensive than plaster. • Follow specific manufacturer's instructions for recommendations on powder-to-water ratios. • A graduated cylinder can be used for measuring water because 1 g of water has a volume very close to 1 mL. • Preweighed envelops of gypsum products are available to eliminate need for weighing. • Stone is often yellow in color, but manufacturers can add colorants to change color of powder.

■ **MATERIAL**

High-Strength Stone (Improved Stone)

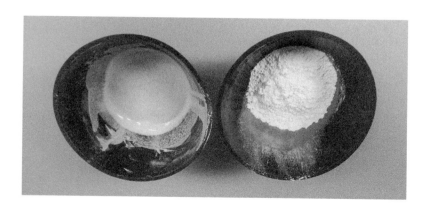

How Supplied ◀ Powder

Composition ◀ Alpha-calcium sulfate hemihydrate

- High-strength or improved stone
- Two flexible mixing bowls
- Mixing spatula
- Water measurer with milliliter markings
- Dental vibrator
- Balance or scale
- Unpoured impression

Directions ▶
1. Measure 100 g of stone and place in first mixing bowl.
2. Measure 19 to 24 mL of room temperature water and place in second mixing bowl.
3. Gradually add preweighed powder to water.
4. Combine powder and water by mixing the two together using mixing spatula.
5. Place mixed stone onto dental vibrator while holding pressure against bowl on dental vibrator.
6. Fill impression using dental vibrator to reduce air bubbles, and allow material to flow into impression.
7. Place filled impression on flat surface away from dental vibrator, and allow to dry.

▶ Special Notes/Helpful Hints • High-strength (improved) stone is the strongest and most expensive gypsum product. • Follow specific manufacturer's instructions for recommendations on powder-to-water ratios. • A graduated cylinder can be used for measuring water because 1 g of water has a volume very close to 1 mL. • Preweighed envelops of gypsum products are available to eliminate need for weighing. • High-strength stone is often supplied in pink, but other colors are available.

Dental Waxes: Pattern and Processing Waxes

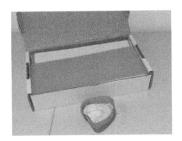

■ MATERIAL Inlay Wax (Pattern Wax)

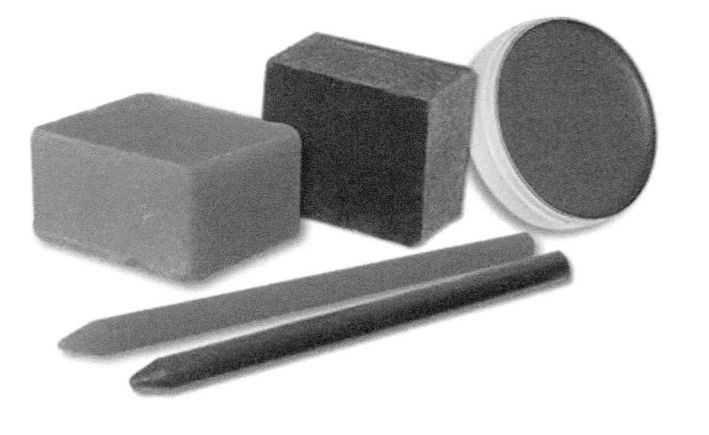

How Supplied ▶ Sticks, pellets, and tins

Composition ▶ Can be a mixture of different waxes, such as paraffin, carnauba, ceresin, and beeswax

• This dental material is used in a dental laboratory setting and arrives to the dental office as a custom order.

Special Notes/Helpful Hints • Inlay wax is used to produce patterns for metal casting through the lost wax technique. • At its working temperature, inlay wax possesses low flow to prevent distortion of the wax pattern. • During the lost wax technique, inlay wax must burn out with no residual because residual material would interfere with casting of the pattern.

MATERIAL Casting Wax (Pattern Wax)

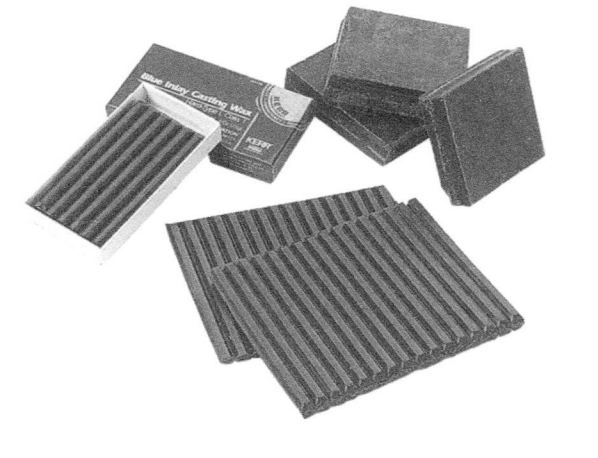

How Supplied ▶ Sheets and preformed shapes

Composition ▶ Can be a mixture of different waxes, such as paraffin, carnauba, ceresin, and beeswax

• This dental material is used in a dental laboratory setting and arrives to the dental office as a custom order.

▐▶ Special Notes/Helpful Hints • Casting wax is used to construct the wax pattern for the metal framework of a partial denture. • Casting wax comes slightly tacky to help hold the material in place on a gypsum cast. • At its working temperature, casting wax possesses low flow to prevent distortion of the wax pattern. • During the lost wax technique, casting wax must burn out with no residual because residual material would interfere with casting of the pattern.

■ MATERIAL Baseplate Wax (Pattern Wax)

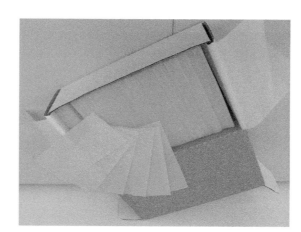

How Supplied ▶ Sheets (7.5 cm wide, 15 cm long, and 0.13 cm thick)

Composition ▶ Ceresin, beeswax, carnauba wax, and various synthetic waxes

• This dental material is used in a dental laboratory setting and arrives to the dental office as a custom order.

◀📖▶ Special Notes/Helpful Hints • Baseplate wax is used to build the contours of a denture and hold the position of the denture teeth before the denture is processed in acrylic. • This material can also be used to take a bite registration for articulation of study casts. • The composition of baseplate wax can be altered to give varying hardness. Examples are as follows: *Type I* is a soft wax at room temperature and is used for contouring a denture. *Type II* is a medium wax that is used for patterns that are placed into the mouth in a temperate climate. *Type III* is a wax with flow qualities at a functioning temperature similar to inlay wax. • Residual stress on the baseplate wax during handling can move teeth and change the occlusion of the denture. • At its working temperature, baseplate wax possesses low flow to prevent distortion of the wax pattern. • During the lost wax technique, casting wax must burn out with no residual because residual material would interfere with casting of the pattern.

■ MATERIAL Boxing Wax (Processing Wax)

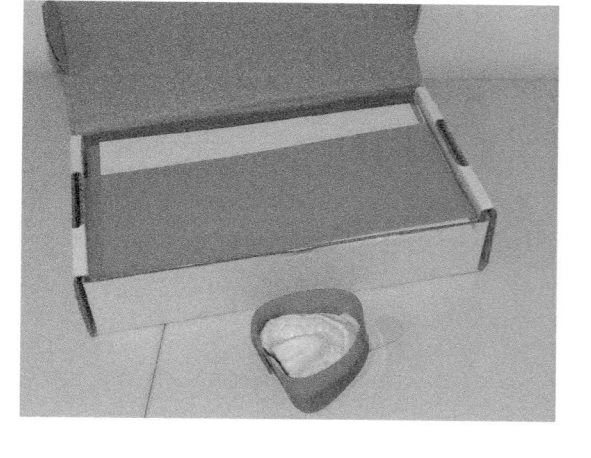

How Supplied ▶ Strips (1 inch, 1.5 inches, and 2 inches)

Composition ▶ Beeswax, paraffin, and other soft waxes

Armamentarium ▶
- Boxing wax
- Stone
- Two flexible mixing bowls
- Mixing spatula
- Water measurer with milliliter markings
- Dental vibrator
- Balance or scale
- Unpoured impression

Directions ▶
1. Mold strip of boxing wax around unpoured impression.
2. Measure 100 g of stone, and place in first mixing bowl.
3. Measure 28 to 32 mL of room temperature water and place in second mixing bowl.
4. Gradually add preweighed powder to water.
5. Combine powder and water by mixing the two together using mixing spatula.
6. Place mixed stone onto dental vibrator while holding pressure against bowl on dental vibrator.
7. Fill impression using dental vibrator to reduce air bubbles and allow material to flow into impression.
8. Place filled impression on flat surface away from dental vibrator and allow to dry.

Special Notes/Helpful Hints • Boxing wax is slightly tacky, which allows the material to attach to stone models, impression trays, or other waxes. • Boxing wax is a pliable wax used primarily in taking and pouring impressions.

■ MATERIAL Utility Wax (Processing Wax)

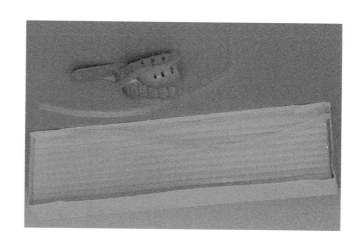

How Supplied ◄ Ropes

Composition ◄ Beeswax, paraffin, and other soft waxes

Armamentarium ▶
- Utility wax
- Impression tray

Directions ▶ Place strips of utility wax along margin or edge of impression tray by squeezing and pushing wax in place.

▶ Special Notes/Helpful Hints • Utility wax is used to reduce irritation of impression tray or soft tissues. • Utility wax can be used to extend the impression tray before taking the impression, and it can help to hold impression material in the impression tray. • Utility wax can be given to orthodontic patients to cover sharp brackets and wires.

MATERIAL ■ Sticky Wax (Processing Wax)

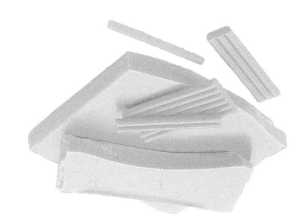

How Supplied ◀ Orange sticks

Composition ◀ Can be a mixture of different waxes, such as paraffin, carnauba, ceresin, and beeswax

• Sticky wax
• Heating element
• Material in need of repair
• Stone model
• Gold carving knife or instrument of choice

1. Place material or appliance needing repair on model.
2. Take gold carving knife or instrument and heat the tip under flame of heating element.
3. Dip heated tip of the instrument into wax, and transfer wax to portion of material or appliance needing repair.
4. Continue to heat instrument, and transfer wax to area of material or appliance needing repair. Wax holds two materials together in proper position while they are sent to dental laboratory for permanent repair.

◀▶ Special Notes/Helpful Hints • Sticky wax is hard and brittle at room temperature and does not become sticky until heated.
• Sticky wax is used to adhere components of metal, gypsum, or resin together temporarily during fabrication and repair. • The dentist may use sticky wax to adhere the two pieces of a broken appliance or some other material together to assist the laboratory in proper repair of the broken appliance.

■ MATERIAL ■ Corrective Impression Wax (Processing Wax)

How Supplied ◄ Wafers or sticks

Composition ◄ Paraffin, ceresin, and castor oil

Armamentarium ▶ • Impression tray
• Impression material
• Corrective impression wax

Directions ▶ 1. Prepare patient for impression of edentulous area.
2. Take impression of edentulous area using impression material of choice.
3. If undercuts are present, place corrective impression wax wafer in first impression.
4. Place impression wax and impression material intraorally simultaneously.
5. Allow impression material to set before removing impression.

◀▶ Special Notes/Helpful Hints • Corrective impression wafers flow at mouth temperature. • Corrective impression sticks must be heated with a heating element to make them malleable. • It is used in conjunction with another impression material to correct undercut areas.

■ **MATERIAL** Bite Registration Wax (Processing Wax)

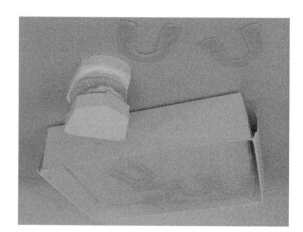

How Supplied ◂ Preformed horseshoe shapes

Composition ◂ Beeswax, paraffin, or ceresin and oils

Armamentarium ▶ • Bite registration wax
• Heating element or hot tap water

Directions ▶ 1. Prepare patient for bite registration.
2. Heat bite registration wax using heating element or hot tap water.
3. When material becomes malleable, place bite registration wax between maxillary and mandibular teeth, and have patient bite lightly.
4. After material has had time to cool completely (about 1 to 2 minutes), remove bite registration wax from patient's mouth and disinfect.

▶ Special Notes/Helpful Hints • Bite registration wax is used to take an impression of how the teeth occlude together. The material takes an impression of the maxillary and mandibular teeth simultaneously. This material is used for accurate articulation of models of opposing arches. • Bite registration wax is susceptible to distortion on removal from the mouth. • Other waxes, such as casting wax or baseplate wax, can be used as bite registration wax. • Addition silicone and polyether materials have replaced waxes for bite registrations.

12

Abrasion, Finishing, and Polishing Materials

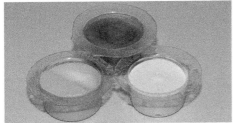

■ **MATERIAL**   Aluminum Oxide

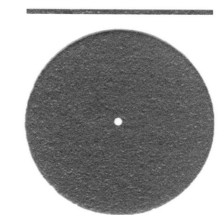

Courtesy Patterson Dental, St. Paul, MN.

How Supplied ◂ Particles attached to discs

Composition ◂ Bauxite

Armamentarium ▶
- Slow-speed handpiece
- Mandrel (screw-type or snap, depending on style of discs)
- Aluminum oxide discs
- Restorative instruments
- Cotton rolls or dental dam

Directions ▶
1. Examine restoration to ensure there are no voids, fractures, or decay.
2. Retract tissues with cotton roll or dental dam.
3. Attach disc containing aluminum oxide to mandrel.
4. Use light, sweeping motion from enamel to restoration.
5. Change order of discs from coarse abrasives to fine abrasives until area being finished and polished is smooth.

◀▶ Special Notes/Helpful Hints • Aluminum oxide is used primarily for finishing and polishing restorations. • Ensure tooth surface is rinsed with water when abrasive discs are changed to prevent more abrasive particles from continuing to abrade surface. • A light, continuous sweeping motion is required to ensure ditching of restoration does not occur. • Tooth surface should be polished with fine polishing paste at conclusion of contouring and polishing with aluminum oxide discs. • Aluminum oxide is red in color. • The material comes in coarse, medium, and fine grits. • Aluminum oxide powders are used in air-abrasion units.

■ MATERIAL   Silicon Carbide

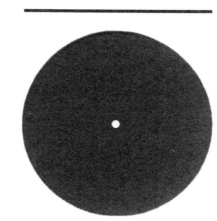

Courtesy Patterson Dental, St. Paul, MN.

How Supplied ▶ Particles attached to discs

Composition ▶ Synthetic material

- Slow-speed handpiece
- Mandrel (screw-type or snap, depending on style of discs)
- Silicon carbide discs
- Restorative instruments
- Cotton rolls or dental dam

Directions ▶
1. Examine restoration to ensure there are no voids, fractures, or decay.
2. Retract tissues with cotton roll or dental dam.
3. Attach disc containing silicon carbide to mandrel.
4. Use light, sweeping motion from enamel to restoration.
5. Change order of discs from course abrasives to fine abrasives until area being polished is smooth.

◀▶ Special Notes/Helpful Hints • Silicon carbide is used primarily for polishing restorations. • Ensure tooth surface is rinsed with water when abrasive discs are changed to prevent more abrasive particles from continuing to abrade surface. • A light, continuous sweeping motion is required to ensure ditching of restoration does not occur. • Tooth surface should be polished with fine polishing paste at conclusion of polishing with silicon carbide discs. • Silicon carbide is black in color. • The material comes in fine, extra-fine, and double-fine grits.

■ MATERIAL ■ Pumice

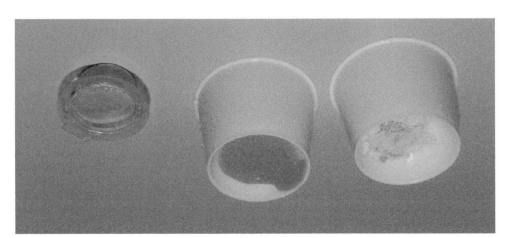

How Supplied ▶ Powder

Composition ▶ Siliceous volcanic glass

• Slow-speed handpiece
• Prophy angle
• Pumice powder
• Dappen dish
• Water or other selected liquid

Directions ▶ 1. Attach prophy angle to slow-speed handpiece, which is connected to dental unit.
2. Place small amount of pumice in Dappen dish, and add small amount of water and mix together with an instrument or the cup of the prophy angle to make a slurry.
3. Place small amount of pumice paste on rubber cup of prophy angle.
4. Dry area to be polished with gauze or compressed air.
5. Press rheostat of dental unit to rotate rubber cup of prophy angle.
6. Place rubber cup of prophy angle loaded with pumice against area to be polished, applying light pressure.

◀▶ Special Notes/Helpful Hints • Pumice is a silica-like volcanic glass used as a polishing agent on enamel, gold foil, and dental amalgam. • Pumice can also be used to finish acrylic denture bases in the dental laboratory. • Pumice can be supplied in premeasured and mixed unit dose cups.

■ **MATERIAL** | Rouge

Courtesy Buffalo Dental Mfg, Syosset, NY.

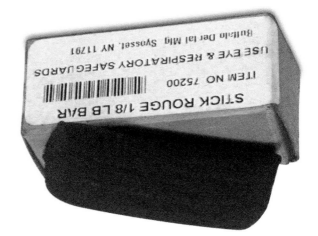

STICK ROUGE 1/8 LB BAR

ITEM NO 75200

USE EYE & RESPIRATORY SAFEGUARDS

Buffalo Dental Mfg. Syosset, NY 11791

How Supplied ◄ Fine red powder pressed into block form

Composition ◄ Iron oxide

- Dental lathe
- Rag wheel
- Rouge

Directions ▶
1. Disinfect appliance being polished according to directions provided by manufacturer for disinfectant.
2. Turn on dental lathe and run block of rouge under rag wheel to cover wheel with rouge.
3. Place area of appliance needing to be polished under rag wheel.
4. Inspect area to see if multiple applications under rag wheel are required. Repeat steps 2 and 3 again until area is smooth.

◀▶ Special Notes/Helpful Hints • Rouge may be impregnated in paper or fabric known as crocus cloth. • Rouge is a polishing agent frequently used in the dental laboratory to polish gold and other noble metal alloys.

■ MATERIAL Cuttle

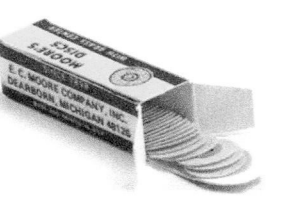

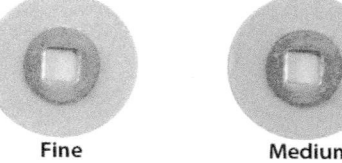

Fine Medium Coarse

How Supplied ▶ Particles bonded to paper

Composition ▶ Quartz

- Slow-speed handpiece
- Mandrel (screw-type or snap, depending on style of discs)
- Cuttle-coated discs
- Restorative instruments
- Cotton rolls or dental dam

Directions ▶
1. Examine restoration and tooth structure to ensure there are no voids, fractures, or decay.
2. Retract tissues with cotton roll or dental dam.
3. Attach coated disc containing cuttle to mandrel.
4. Use light, sweeping motion from enamel to restoration.
5. Change order of discs from course abrasives to fine abrasives until area being polished is smooth.

◀▶ Special Notes/Helpful Hints • Ensure tooth surface is rinsed with water when abrasive discs are changed to prevent more abrasive particles from continuing to abrade surface. • A light, continuous sweeping motion is required to ensure ditching of restoration does not occur. • The tooth surface should be polished with fine polishing paste at the conclusion of polishing with cuttle discs. • Cuttle is beige in color and supplied in course, medium, and fine grits. • The cuttlebone mounted in a bird's cage is made of the same material.

■ **MATERIAL** Garnet

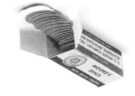

Courtesy E.C. Moore Co., Inc., Dearborn, MI.

Xtra-Fine   Fine   Medium   Coarse

How Supplied ◄ Mixture of ground minerals attached to coated discs

Composition ◄ Oxides of aluminum iron and silicon

• Slow-speed handpiece
• Mandrel (screw-type or snap, depending on style of discs)
• Garnet-coated discs
• Restorative instruments
• Cotton rolls or dental dam

Directions ▶ 1. Examine restoration and tooth structure to ensure there are no voids, fractures, or decay.
2. Retract tissues with cotton roll or dental dam.
3. Attach coated disc containing garnet to mandrel.
4. Use light, sweeping motion from enamel to restoration.
5. Change order of discs from course abrasives to fine abrasives until area being polished is smooth.

◀▶ Special Notes/Helpful Hints • Ensure tooth surface is rinsed with water when abrasive discs are changed to prevent more abrasive particles from continuing to abrade surface. • A light continuous sweeping motion is required to ensure ditching of restoration does not occur. • The tooth surface should be polished with fine polishing paste at conclusion of polishing with garnet discs. • Garnet is usually dark red in color and available in extra-coarse, coarse, medium, fine, and extra-fine grits. • Garnet is used for grinding plastics and metal alloys.

■ **MATERIAL** Emery

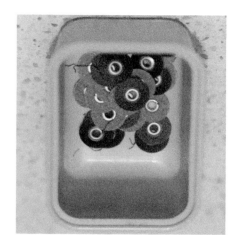

How Supplied ◄ Powder attached to disc

Composition ◄ Corundum

Armamentarium ▶
- Slow-speed handpiece
- Mandrel (screw-type or snap, depending on style of discs)
- Emery-coated discs
- Restorative instruments
- Cotton rolls or dental dam

Directions ▶
1. Examine restoration and tooth structure to ensure there are no voids, fractures, or decay.
2. Retract tissues with cotton roll or dental dam.
3. Attach coated disc containing emery to mandrel.
4. Use light, sweeping motion from enamel to restoration.

▶ Special Notes/Helpful Hints • Emery often is used to smooth or reshape the surface of the tooth, such as the incisal edge.
• Emery resembles grayish black sand. • Emery can be used intraorally or in the dental laboratory with a dental lathe. • This is the same material used on emery boards to file fingernails.

■ **MATERIAL** Silex

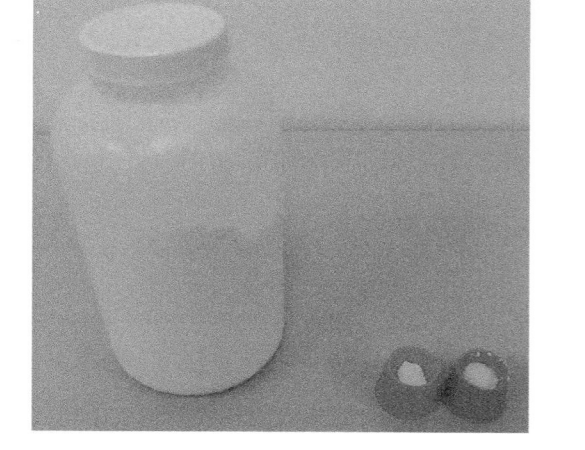

How Supplied ▶ Powder

Composition ▶ Quartz or tripoli

• Slow-speed handpiece
- Prophy angle
- Silex powder
- Dappen dish
- Water or other selected liquid

1. Attach prophy angle to slow-speed handpiece, which is connected to dental unit.
2. Place small amount of silex in Dappen dish, and add small amount of water and mix together with an instrument or the cup of the prophy angle to make a slurry.
3. Place small amount of silex paste on rubber cup of prophy angle.
4. Dry area to be polished with gauze or compressed air.
5. Press rheostat of dental unit to rotate rubber cup of prophy angle.
6. Place rubber cup of prophy angle loaded with silex paste against area or restoration to be polished, applying light pressure.

◀▶ Special Notes/Helpful Hints • Silex is used as an abrasive agent to polish restorations.

■ **MATERIAL** Tin Oxide

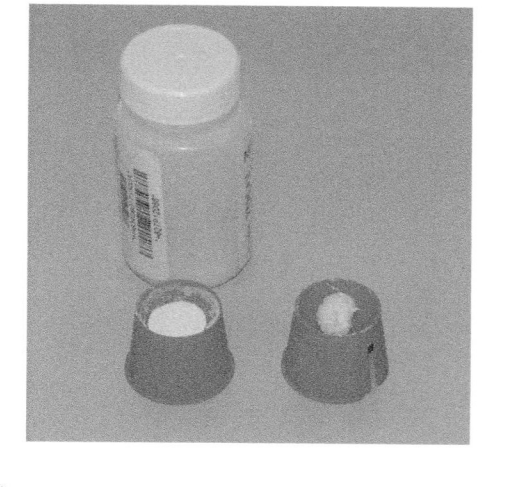

How Supplied ▶ White powder

Composition ▶ Tin oxide

• Slow-speed handpiece
- Prophy angle
- White tin oxide powder
- Dappen dish
- Water

Directions ▶ 1. Attach prophy angle to slow-speed handpiece, which is connected to dental unit.
2. Place small amount of tin oxide in Dappen dish, and add small amount of water and mix together with an instrument or the cup of the prophy angle to make a slurry.
3. Place small amount of tin oxide paste on rubber cup of prophy angle.
4. Dry area to be polished with gauze or compressed air.
5. Press rheostat of dental unit to rotate rubber cup of prophy angle.
6. Place rubber cup of prophy angle loaded with tin oxide paste against area or restoration to be polished, applying light pressure.

◀▶ Special Notes/Helpful Hints • Tin oxide is used as a final polishing agent for teeth and metallic restorations. • Tin oxide can be mixed with water, alcohol, or glycerin.

■ **MATERIAL**   Prophy Paste (Pumice)

How Supplied ◄ Unit-dose cups; variety of colors, textures, flavors, grits, and formulations

Composition ◄ Pumice and additives

Armamentarium ▶
- Slow-speed handpiece
- Prophy angle
- Unit-dose prophy paste

Directions ▶
1. Attach prophy angle to slow-speed handpiece, which is connected to dental unit.
2. Select appropriate prophy paste for area to be polished.
3. Place small amount of prophy paste on rubber cup of prophy angle.
4. Dry area to be polished with gauze or compressed air.
5. Press rheostat of dental unit to rotate rubber cup of prophy angle.
6. Place rubber cup of prophy angle loaded with prophy paste against area or restoration to be polished, applying light pressure.

◀▶ Special Notes/Helpful Hints • Prophy pastes should create a high polish of the tooth surface or restoration without extensively abrading the surface. • All abrasives in prophy pastes break down into smaller and smaller particles during the polishing procedure. • Calcium carbonate is found in prophy paste and dentifrices. It is also known as chalk or whiting. • Some prophy pastes contain fluoride.

Specialty Materials

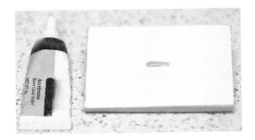

■ **MATERIAL**

CAD/CAM Restoration—Digital Impression

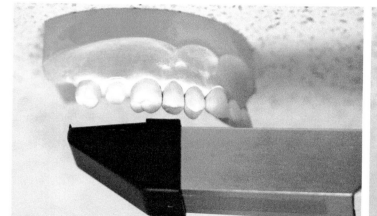 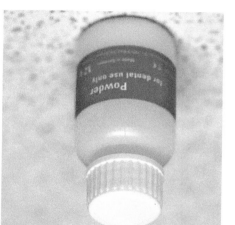

How Supplied ► Powder

Composition ► Blue antireflective contrast medium

- Restorative instruments
- CAD/CAM system with optical scanner
- CAD/CAM impression powder

Directions ▶
1. Prepare tooth for an indirect restoration.
2. Clean tooth with water, and isolate it to prevent contamination during impression.
3. Coat prepared tooth lightly with impression powder (blue antireflective contrast medium), ensuring all surfaces of prepared tooth and adjacent areas are coated.
4. Place optical scanner over prepared tooth. When scanner is in correct position and image quality is good, capture image and upload into computer.
5. Design restoration on computer, and cut from solid block of porcelain in separate milling unit.

◀▶ Special Notes/Helpful Hints • The CAD/CAM camera that takes the optical impression measures the dimensions of the tooth structure. Applying excessive amounts of powder to the tooth surface can distort the optical impression.

▪ MATERIAL Topical Fluoride

How Supplied ▶ Foam and gel

Composition ▶ Acidulated phosphate or sodium fluoride and flavoring agents

• Topical fluoride
• Fluoride tray

• Saliva ejector
• Gauze squares

Directions ▶ 1. Assess patient for type of fluoride to apply to tooth surface.
   • Neutral fluoride should be used for patients who have ceramic or composite restorations.
   • Acidulated phosphate fluoride should be used on patients without restorations or with restorations containing only metal.
2. Select fluoride, and apply a thin strip into appropriate size fluoride tray.
3. Dry tooth surfaces with gauze square or compressed air.
4. Place fluoride trays intraorally, squeezing trays around teeth to extrude material into interproximal surfaces.
5. Give patient saliva ejector to hold and place in mouth to suction excess saliva out of mouth.
6. Remove fluoride trays at conclusion of treatment, and allow patient to suction remaining material from mouth.

◀▶ Special Notes/Helpful Hints • Different fluoride products can be applied to the tooth surface for 1 to 4 minutes. Research has indicated the 4-minute application is the most effective. • The patient should be given instructions *not* to close around the saliva ejector while the fluoride trays are in place because this can cause negative pressure and suck back in the vacuum line, and bacteria in the vacuum line can come back into the patient's mouth causing cross-contamination. Some vacuum lines have a system that prevents negative pressure. • Acidulated phosphate fluorides can etch ceramic and composite, and this type of fluoride is not recommended for patients with such restorations.

■ **MATERIAL** Fluoride Varnish

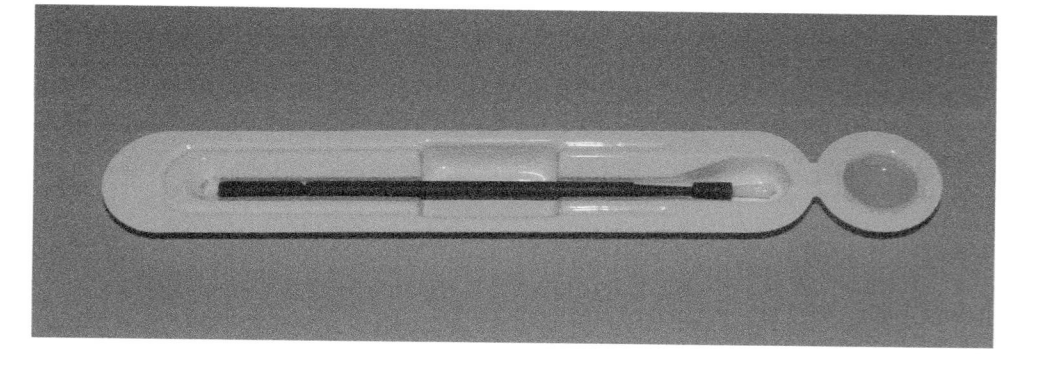

How Supplied ▶ Paste

Composition ▶ Sodium fluoride

Armamentarium ▶
- Fluoride varnish
- Disposable applicator brush
- Dappen dish
- Disposable cup

Directions ▶
1. Remove excessive amounts of saliva from mouth and tooth structure where fluoride varnish is to be placed.
2. Dip disposable applicator brush into fluoride varnish and paint varnish on facial and lingual surfaces of tooth according to manufacturer's instructions.
3. Instruct patient to spit in disposable cup to remove excessive amounts of saliva from oral cavity.

◀▶ Special Notes/Helpful Hints • Some fluoride varnishes require application to both the facial and the lingual surfaces, whereas others require application to only one side of the tooth surface. Read manufacturer's instructions before use. • Fluoride varnishes creep into the interproximal surfaces of the teeth and remain on the tooth surface for 4 to 6 hours after placement. • Post-treatment instructions should be given to a patient after a fluoride varnish treatment. Most manufacturers supply post-treatment patient care instructions, which can be sent home with the patient at the conclusion of the treatment. • Do not suction fluoride varnish out of a patient's mouth with the saliva ejector because the material can accumulate on the sides of the suction hose and cause the hose to become blocked. Instead, a disposable cup should be used during the application process.

MATERIAL Sealant

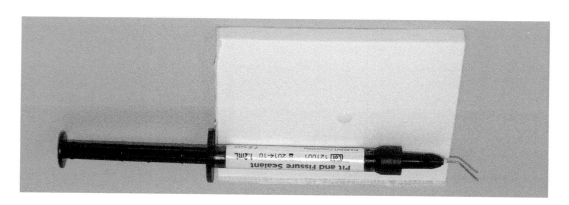

How Supplied ▶ Syringe

Composition ▶ Resin

- Sealant
- Etchant
- Primer (when indicated)
- Curing light
- Shepard's hook explorer
- Low-speed or slow-speed handpiece
- Prophy angle with brush tip
- Dappen dish
- Pumice
- Isolation materials (rubber dam, dry angles, cotton rolls, gauze squares)

Directions ▶
1. Isolate tooth surface being sealed with use of rubber dam or other means.
2. Clean tooth surface with slurry of pumice.
3. Rinse and dry tooth surface thoroughly.
4. Etch tooth surface with 37% orthophosphoric acid.

Cont'd Directions ▶
5. Rinse with water.
6. Dry tooth surface and place sealant material.
7. Polymerize sealant material with curing light.
8. Assess tooth surface with explorer to ensure that all pits and fissures are covered, no voids are present, and sealant is well retained.
9. Apply more material, if needed.
10. Remove isolation and check occlusion, making adjustments where needed.
11. Check contacts with floss.

• Filler particle size can vary among sealants. Some sealants have small filler particles, and other materials have no filler particles. • The color of the sealant material can vary. Some sealants are white, and other materials are clear. Isolation during sealant placement is essential for success and longevity of the sealant. Isolation materials may require replacement as they become saturated throughout the procedure when a rubber dam cannot be used. • Some manufacturers recommend use of a primer before placement of a sealant when a rubber dam cannot be used for isolation. The primer is believed to help the sealant wet a slightly contaminated area.

Formocresol

How Supplied ▶ Liquid

Composition ▶ Formaldehyde, cresol, and glycerin

• Restorative instruments
• Rubber dam
• Formocresol
• Dappen dish
• Cotton pliers
• Cotton pellets
• Gauze squares

Directions ▶ 1. Isolate tooth requiring endodontic treatment with rubber dam.
2. Clean, debride, and instrument canals.
3. Rinse and dry canal spaces.
4. Moisten cotton pellets with formocresol and blot excess liquid from pellets with gauze.
5. Place cotton pellets in pulp chamber, and seal access hole with temporary filling material.
6. Recall patient after a minimum of 48 hours to remove pellets.
7. Complete endodontic treatment.

▶ Special Notes/Helpful Hints • Formocresol is used as a disinfectant and devitalizing solution as part of endodontic treatment.
• The material can also be used for pulpotomy by placing formocresol pellets on remaining radicular pulp for 5 minutes. After the 5-minute application, remove pellets and restore tooth with base or core material.

■ MATERIAL Gutta Percha

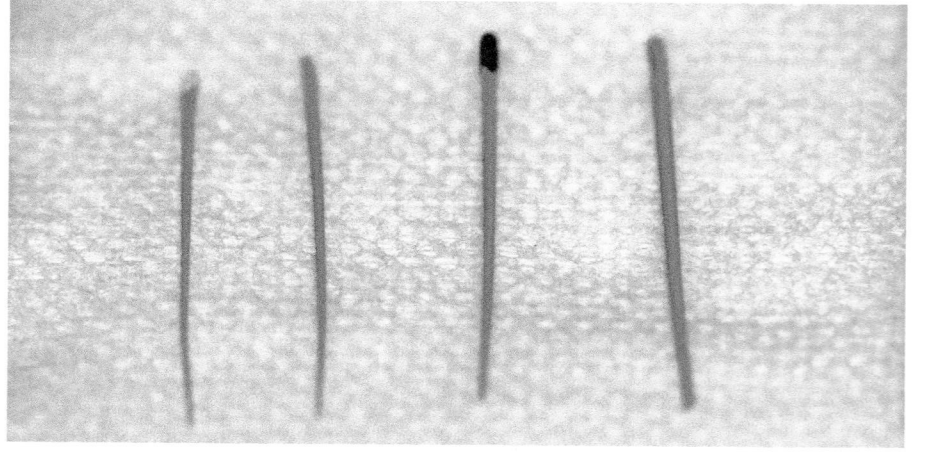

How Supplied ▶ Cylindrical points

Composition ▶ Natural rubber

Armamentarium ▶
- Restorative instruments
- Endodontic instruments
- Heat source
- Rubber dam
- Cotton pliers

Directions ▶
1. Isolate tooth needing endodontic treatment with rubber dam.
2. Clean, debride, and instrument canals.
3. Rinse and dry canal spaces.
4. Select appropriate size gutta percha points for diameter of each canal being filled.
5. Pull tip of gutta percha through root canal sealing material and place gutta percha point in appropriate canal.
6. Heat endodontic instruments and condense gutta percha into canal.
7. Remove excess material after heating and seal access hole with restorative material.

◀▶ Special Notes/Helpful Hints • Gutta percha is used to obturate canals after endodontic treatment. • Gutta percha becomes plastic on heating and is very resistant to water.

■ MATERIAL   Root Canal Sealer

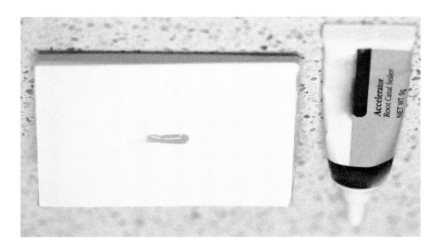

How Supplied ◄ Paste

Composition ◄ Calcium hydroxide and fillers

Armamentarium ▶ • Restorative instruments
- Endodontic instruments
- Heat source
- Rubber dam
- Cotton pliers

Directions ▶ 1. Isolate tooth needing endodontic treatment with rubber dam.
2. Clean, debride, and instrument canals.
3. Rinse and dry canal spaces.
4. Select appropriate size gutta percha points for diameter of each canal being filled.
5. Place small amount of root canal sealer on mixing pad.
6. Pull tip of gutta percha through root canal sealing material and place gutta percha point in appropriate canal.
7. Heat endodontic instruments and condense gutta percha into canal.
8. Remove excess material after heating and seal access hole with restorative material.

◀▶ Special Notes/Helpful Hints • Gutta percha is used to fill the canal after endodontic treatment, whereas root canal sealer is used to seal the opening at the apex of the root that has undergone endodontic treatment. Sealing the apex is a means to prevent bacteria from reentering the canals of the tooth.

MATERIAL ■ Root Canal Lubricant

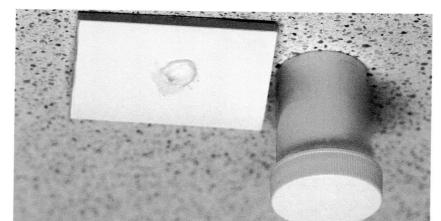

How Supplied ▶ Paste

Composition ▶ Glycol and peroxide

Armamentarium ▶
- Restorative instruments
- Endodontic instruments
- Rubber dam
- Cotton pliers

Directions ▶
1. Isolate tooth needing endodontic treatment with rubber dam.
2. Place small amount of root canal lubricant on wax mixing pad or 2×2 gauze square.
3. Clean, debride, and instrument canals by dipping endodontic files in root canal lubricant and moving files up and down canals of tooth being treated.
4. Continue this process until all infected tissue has been removed from canals.
5. Rinse and dry canal spaces.
6. Complete endodontic treatment.

◀▣▶ Special Notes/Helpful Hints • Root canal lubricant is used to make the process of instrumenting canals of a tooth with the endodontic files easier. • The material also has an effervescent action, which brings bacteria and debris coronally during instrumentation of the canals. • Some manufacturers have root canal lubricant in single-dose applications that can be dispensed directly into the canal of the tooth being treated.

■ **MATERIAL**

Periodontal Dressing

How Supplied ◀ Two pastes

Composition ◀ Calcium sulfate, zinc oxide, polymethyl methacrylate, and flavoring

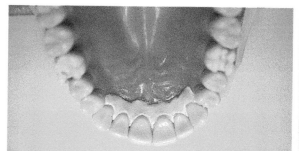

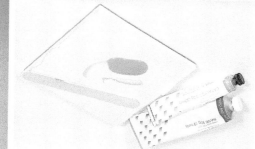

From Hatrick, Eakle, and Bird, 2011.

• Periodontal dressing material
- Spatula
- Large mixing pad

Directions ▶ 1. Extrude equal lengths of paste from each tube of material.
2. Spatulate material together until two pastes are uniform in color.
3. Use spatula to form cylindrical shape with material.
4. Lubricate fingers with petroleum jelly (Vaseline), lanolin, cold cream, or water.
5. With fingers lubricated, roll material with fingertips off of mixing pad.
6. Shape material into ropes to be shaped against tissue and teeth.

◀▶ Special Notes/Helpful Hints • Some patients may have an allergy or sensitivity to some components of the periodontal dressing material. Do not use on a patient with a history of this allergy or sensitivity.

■ **MATERIAL** | Alveolar Dressing

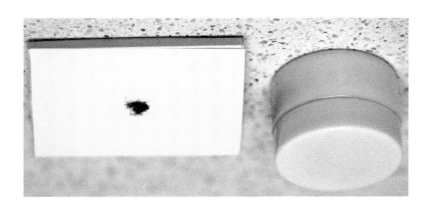

How Supplied ◄ Paste

Composition ◄ Eugenol, sodium lauryl sulfate, and calcium carbonate

Armamentarium ▶
- Restorative or extraction instruments
- Cotton pliers
- Mixing pad

Directions ▶
1. Dispense small amount of paste onto mixing pad.
2. Take small pellet of paste and place gently into prepared dental socket with cotton pliers. (Do not suture.)
3. Instruct patient not to wash mouth out vigorously for 24 hours after extraction or placement of alveolar dressing.

◀▶ Special Notes/Helpful Hints • Alveolar dressing material is used to treat a dry socket after an extraction. • The material can be placed after a traumatic extraction or in a socket of a patient with a history of dry socket. • Some patients may have an allergy or sensitivity to some components of the alveolar dressing material. Do not use on a patient with a history of this allergy or sensitivity.

Historical Dental Materials

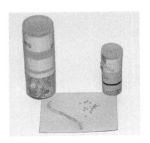

■ MATERIAL Low-Copper Dental Amalgam

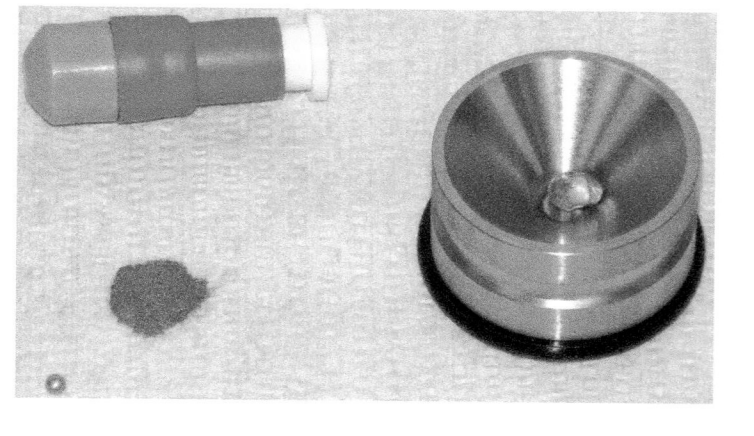

How Supplied ▶ Capsules

Composition ▶ Silver, copper, tin, and liquid mercury

- Amalgam capsule
- Amalgamator
- Amalgam well
- Amalgam carrier
- Restorative instruments
- Cotton roll
- Tofflemire and matrix band (if restoration is a class II)

Directions ▶

1. Activate amalgam restorative material capsule by squeezing two ends of capsule together, if indicated by manufacturer.
2. Place capsule in amalgamator and triturate for time indicated, according to manufacturer's instructions.
3. Dry area where restoration is to be placed and keep area isolated.
4. Place mixed amalgam in amalgam well.
5. Load amalgam carrier with mixed amalgam and carry amalgam to prepared tooth structure.
6. Place material into prepared tooth structure.
7. Using condenser, press and condense amalgam into prepared tooth structure.
8. Continue to load prepared tooth with amalgam while condensing material into prepared tooth structure.

▶ Cont'd Directions

9. When prepared tooth structure has been overfilled with amalgam and all material has been condensed or packed into prepared tooth structure, begin carving and shaping of restoration.
10. Burnish outer surface of restoration with a football or ball burnisher.
11. Carve away excess material with a Hollenback carver, Wedelstadt chisel, or other instrument of choice.
12. Burnish amalgam again with football or ball burnisher, or use acorn burnisher to place grooves into surface of amalgam.
13. Wet a cotton roll, and rub cotton roll over surface of amalgam to remove excess material remaining from carving.

If the prepared tooth is a class II preparation, a matrix band must be used to maintain the shape of the restoration during placement. The matrix band should be placed before activation or trituration of amalgam. Amalgam does not fully set-up until 24 hours after placement. Final polishing or adjustment should not occur for a minimum of 24 hours.

• Low-copper dental amalgam is no longer used in clinical practice. This material is also known as traditional or conventional amalgam. • Amalgams with more than 1% zinc are considered zinc-containing amalgam. Clinical research shows zinc-containing amalgam has a longer clinical life expectancy than nonzinc amalgam.

■ MATERIAL Direct Gold Restorative Materials

How Supplied ▶ Foil or pellets

Composition ▶ Gold and wax

- Restorative instruments
- Alcohol torch
- Gold placement instrument
- Rubber dam

Directions ▶
1. Place rubber dam to isolate area where tooth is being restored.
2. Prepare tooth for restoration.
3. Rinse and dry preparation thoroughly.
4. Place base material, if needed.
5. Using placement instrument, place pellet of gold on top of alcohol flame to burn off wax.
6. Carefully place pellet of gold in preparation using a condenser to push it gently into place.
7. Condense material with condenser to ensure no air space is remaining.
8. Continue to place and condense gold restorative material until prepared tooth structure is filled.
9. Use beaver-tail burnisher to smooth outer surface of restorative material. Burnish in the direction from gold to tooth.
10. Discoid cleoid or sandpaper disc can be used to remove excess material.
11. Polish to smooth surface with rubber cup and aluminum oxide.

◀▶ Special Notes/Helpful Hints • Pure metals are seldom used in dentistry because they lack properties that make them useful intraorally. • Direct gold restorations historically were used for small class I and class IV restorations.

■ **MATERIAL** Agar: Reversible Hydrocolloid

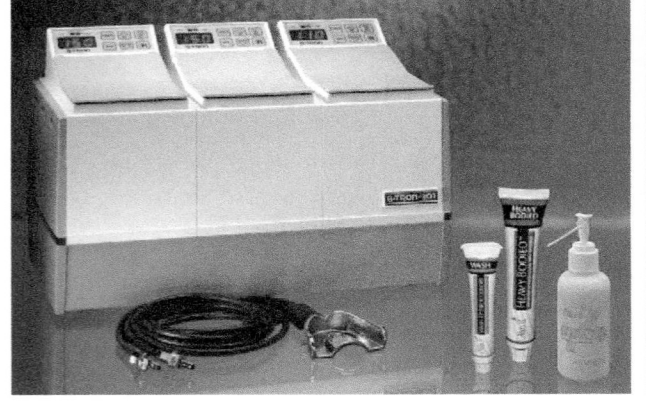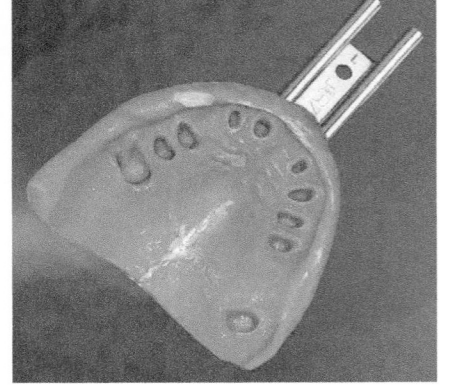

Courtesy Dux Dental, Oxnard, CA.

How Supplied ▶ Semisolid material in tubes and sticks

Composition ▶ Agar, potassium sulfate, borax, alkyl benzoate, and water

• Hydrocolloid conditioner
- Hydrocolloid impression trays
- Cooling hoses
- Hydrocolloid impression material

Directions ▶
1. Boil hydrocolloid impression material in first compartment of hydrocolloid conditioner.
2. Store prepared hydrocolloid material in middle compartment of hydrocolloid conditioner (prepared materials can be stored for several days). Water in this compartment should be 150° F.
3. Select appropriate size tray to take impression, and attach cooling hoses.
4. Temper hydrocolloid material by placing it in third compartment (far right). Water in this compartment should be at least 110° F. (It is essential to reduce the temperature of the agar material to ensure the oral tissues do not get burned.)
5. Place hydrocolloid material in impression trays and place trays in patient's mouth, ensuring cool water is running through the cooling hoses attached to the impression trays.

◀▶ Special Notes/Helpful Hints • Agar has a special characteristic known as hysteresis. Hysteresis refers to when a material melts and gels at different temperatures. • Agar melts at a much higher temperature (boiling) and gels at mouth temperature.

Glossary

A

Abrasive – Material that wears or abrades another material.

Adhesion – Act of sticking two items together. In dentistry, the bonding or cementation process.

Adhesive – Material that causes two materials to stick together.

Alginate – Irreversible hydrocolloid impression material.

Alloy – Mixture of two or more metals.

Amalgam – Mixture of metal alloy with liquid mercury.

Armamentarium – Equipment and supplies needed to manipulate dental materials.

B

Base – Layer of material, usually cement, that acts as an insulator and protective barrier under a restoration.

Biocompatible – Property of dental materials that prevents a material from adversely affecting living tissue.

C

Cast – Replica of a patient's intraoral structures; made of gypsum material.

Contamination – Contact with a material, such as saliva, that prevents a dental material from setting appropriately.

Corrosive – Acid or strong base that can cause damage to skin, clothing, metals, and equipment.

Creep – Small change in the shape of a restoration; caused by continuous compression from occlusion or adjacent teeth.

Custom-made – Appliance or other instrument used in dentistry that is made specifically to fit one individual.

D

Denture base – Usually pink-colored; material used to support artificial teeth that sits on the alveolar ridge.

Dual-cure materials – Materials that set by a dual reaction.

E

Elastomers – Highly accurate elastic impression materials that have qualities similar to rubber.

Endodontic files – Instruments used to remove contents of root canal and to shape root canal to receive filling material such as gutta percha.

Etch – Process of preparing a tooth surface for bonding.

Eugenol – Organic liquid that is the major component of oil of cloves. It is antibacterial and obtundent to the pulp.

Exothermic reaction – Production of heat resulting from the reactions of some dental materials when they are mixed together.

F

Final set time – Time from the start of the mix until the material becomes rigid.

Finishing – Procedure used to give a restoration its final shape and contour.

G

Glass ionomer – Restorative material containing fluoride; used to restore tooth structure or as a cement.

Gypsum – Material found in nature comprising calcium sulfate hemihydrate; used to make dental casts and dies and to attach models to articulators.

H

Hazardous chemicals – Chemicals that can be dangerous or poisonous that can cause bodily harm or fire.

Homogeneous – Material having a smooth consistent appearance.

I

Impression – Negative copy.

L

Lost wax casting technique – Procedure used to fabricate a metal restoration by encasing a wax pattern in stone and then vaporizing the wax under high temperatures to leave an empty impression space (pattern) previously occupied by the wax. Molten metal is cast into the space and takes the shape of the pattern.

M

Margin – Junction of the tooth and the restoration that is visible clinically.

Mixing time – Amount of time required to bring the components of a material together into a homogeneous mix.

O

Obtundent – The quality of soothing the pulp of the tooth when discomfort occurs as a result of the removal of decay.

P

Personal protection equipment – Equipment worn by an employee that provides protection during clinical and laboratory procedures.

Polishing – Procedure that produces a shiny, smooth surface by eliminating fine scratches, minor surface irregularities, surface stains, and debris such as plaque by using mild abrasives.

Polymerization – Act of forming polymers; a term used frequently to describe the setting or curing of composites or resins.

Polymers – Materials made of large, long molecules formed by chemically reacting molecular building blocks called monomers.

Porosity – Multiple microscopic holes or voids in a material.

Prosthesis – Appliance used to replace missing teeth and tissues.

Provisional – Temporary restoration that covers the prepared tooth structure and takes the place of a permanent restoration while the permanent restoration is being fabricated.

R

Resin-modified glass ionomer – Restorative material containing resin and fluoride; used to restore tooth structure or as a cement.

S

Silane coupling agent – Chemical that helps to bind filler particles to the polymer matrix.

Sol – Liquid state in which colloidal particles are suspended.

Solubility – Susceptible to being dissolved.

Stropping – To mix a material by flipping a spatula from side to side and whipping vigorously.

V

Viscous – Description for material when it is thick and has high resistance to flow.

W

Working time – Amount of time from the start of the mix until the material reaches a semihard state.

Appendix A Conversion Tables

Temperature

Celsius (° C) = 5/9 Fahrenheit (° F) − 32

Fahrenheit (° F) = 9/5 Celsius (° C) + 32

Linear Measurement

Metric

1 meter (m) = 100 centimeters (cm)

1 centimeter (cm) = 0.01 meter (m)

1 millimeter (mm) = 0.001 meter (m)

1 micrometer (μm*) = 0.001 millimeter (mm)

1 nanometer (nm) = 0.000001 mm

1 angstrom (Å) = 0.0000001 mm

Converting U.S. (English) Measurements to Metric

1 inch (in) = 25.4 millimeters (mm) = 2.54 centimeters (cm)

39.37 inches (in) = 1 meter (m)

*Also called micron.

3.28 feet (ft) = 1 meter (m)

1 yard (yd) = 0.9144 meter (m)

Liquid Measurement

Metric

1 liter (L) = 1000 milliliters (mL) = 1000 cubic centimeters (cm³)

Converting U.S. (English) Measurements to Metric

1 quart (qt) = 0.946 liter (L)

1 ounce (oz) = 29.6 milliliters (mL)

Weight

Metric

1 kilogram (kg) = 1000 grams (g)

1 gram (g) = 0.001 kilogram (kg) = 1,000,000 micrograms (µg)

1 milligram (mg) = 0.001 gram (g)

Converting Metric to U.S. (English) Measurements

1 kilogram (kg) = 2.2 pounds (lb)

1 gram (g) = 0.0022 pound (lb) = 0.035 ounce (oz)

28.35 gram (g) = 1 ounce (oz)

Common Measures of Weight for Gold
1 troy ounce (oz) = 20 pennyweight (dwt)
1 pennyweight = 1.555 grams (g) = 24 grains (gr)
1 grain (gr) = 0.065 gram (g)

Measures of Gold Content
24 carat = 100% gold = 1000 fine
12 carat = 50% gold = 500 fine

Measures of Force (per Area)
1 kilogram/square centimeter $(kg/cm^2) = 14.223$ pounds/square inch (lb/in^2)
1 $kg/cm^2 = 0.0981$ megapascals (MPa)
1 meganewton/square meter $(MN/m^2) = 145$ lb/in^2

Appendix B Commonly Used Trade Materials

Varnish

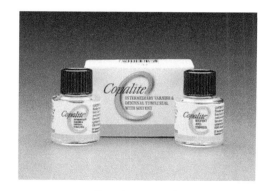

Copalite varnish
Cooley & Cooley, Ltd.

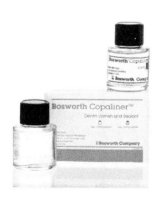

Bosworth Copaliner varnish
Harry J. Bosworth Company

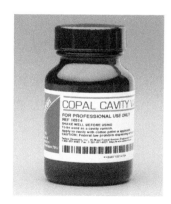

Copal Cavity Varnish
Sultan Healthcare

Calcium Hydroxide Low Strength Base

Calcimol LC calcium hydroxide paste
VOCO America, Inc.

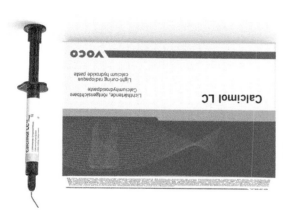

Dycal Calcium Hydroxide
Composition cavity lining material
DENTSPLY Caulk

Bosworth Hydrox Calcium
Hydroxide Paste cavity liner
Harry J. Bosworth Company

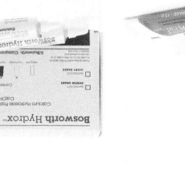

Glass Ionomer "Light Cure" High Strength Base

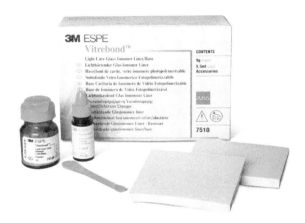

Vitrebon Light Cure Glass Ionomer Liner/Base
3M ESPE Dental Products

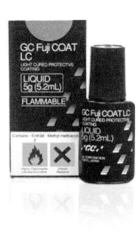

GC Fuji COAT LC Light Cured
Protective Coating glass ionomer
GC America Inc.

TheraCal LC
Bisco, Inc.

Resin-Modified Calcium Silicate High Strength Base

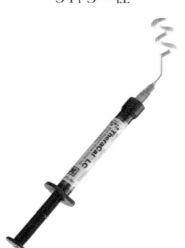

Vitrebond Plus Light Cure Glass Ionomer Liner/Base
3M ESPE Dental Products

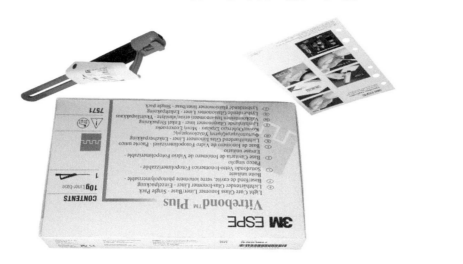

3M ESPE

Vitrebond™ Plus

Light Cure Glass Ionomer Liner/Base - Single Pack
Lichthärtender Glas-Ionomer Liner - Einzelpackung
Base/fond de cavité, verre ionomère photopolymérisable -
Boîte unitaire
Sonucdoban Veto-Ionomérico Fotopolimerizzabile -
Pacco singolo
Base Cavitaria de Ionómero de Vidrio Fotopolimerizable -
Envase unitario
Base de Ionómero de Vidro Fotopolimerizável - Pacote único
Lichthärtend Glas Ionomeer Liner - Enkelverpakking
Φωτοπολυμεριζόμενη Υαλοïονομερής
Κονιο/Οδοντρο Χρωσια - Μονη Συσκευασια
Lyshærdende Glasionomer Liner - Enkeltpakning
Valokovetteva Iasi-ionomeri etoe/alusaine - Yksittäispakkaus
Lyshärdande Glasjonomer Liner - Enkelpakning
Lyshærdende glasionomer liner/base - Single pack

CONTENTS
10g Liner-base   1

7571

Etchant

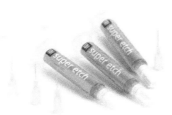

Super Etch
SDI Limited

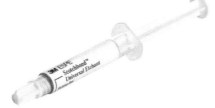

Scotchbond Universal Etchant
3M ESPE Dental Products

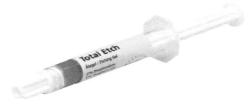

Total Etch
Ivoclar Vivadent Inc.

Total Etch Bonding Agent

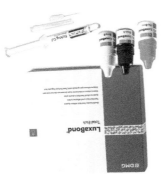

iBond Total Etch
Heraeus Kulzer, LLC

Clearfil DC Bond dental bonding agent
Kuraray America, Inc.

LuxaBond Total Etch
intro kit
DMG America

Self-Etching Bonding Agent

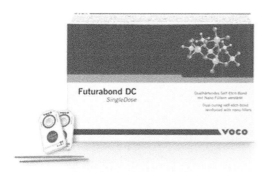

Futurabond DC
VOCO America, Inc.

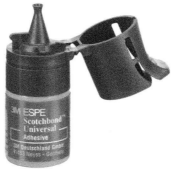

Scotchbond Universal Adhesive
3M ESPE Dental Products

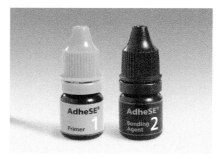

AdheSE
Ivoclar Vivadent Inc.

Admix High Copper Amalgam

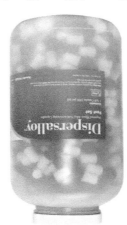

Dispersalloy Dispersed Phase Alloy Self-Activating
Capsules
DENTSPLY Caulk

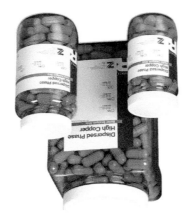

Royale Dispersed Phase High Copper Dental
Amalgam Alloy
DMG America

Spherical High-Copper Amalgam

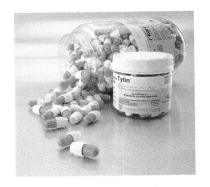

Tytin amalgam capsules
Kerr Corporation

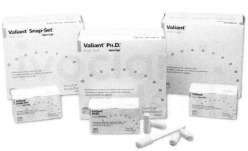

Valiant Sure-Cap packs
Ivoclar Vivadent Inc.

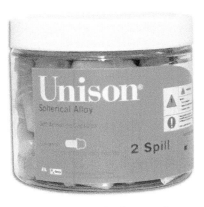

Unison Spherical Alloy amalgam
DENTSPLY Caulk

Macrofilled Composite

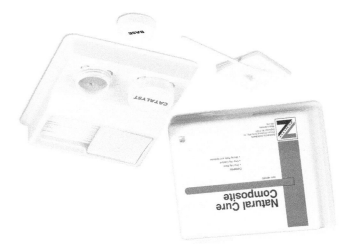

Natural Cure Composite
DMG America

Microfilled Composite

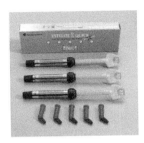

Estelite Sigma Quick
Tokuyama Dental
Corporation Inc.

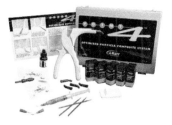

Point 4 Optimized Particle
Composite System
Kerr Corporation

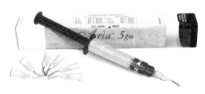

Aria Microfill Flowable Composite
Danville Materials

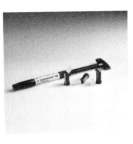

Heliomolar HB flow
composite material
Ivoclar Vivadent Inc.

Hybrid Composite

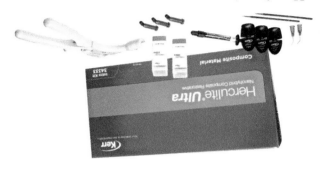

Herculite Ultra Nanohybrid Composite Restorative
Kerr Corporation

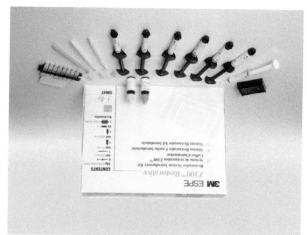

Z100 Restorative
3M ESPE Dental Products

Improved Hybrid Composite

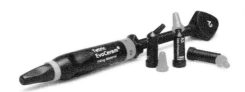

Tetric EvoCeram
Ivoclar Vivadent Inc.

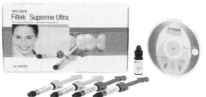

Filtek Supreme Ultra
3M ESPE Dental Products

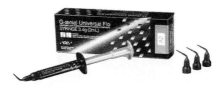

G-ænial Universal Flo
GC America Inc.

Flowable Composite

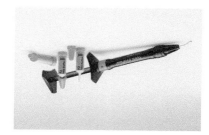

Tetric EvoFlow
Ivoclar Vivadent Inc.

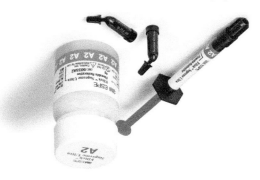

Filtek Supreme Ultra Flowable Restorative
3M ESPE Dental Products

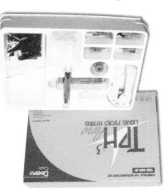

TPH³flow Liquid Micro
Hybrid flowable composite
DENTSPLY Caulk

Resin Modified Glass Ionomer Restorative Material

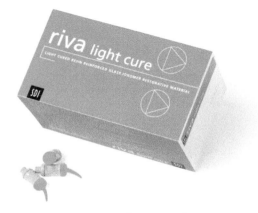

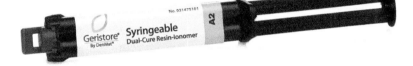

Riva Light Cure Glass
Ionomer Restorative Material
SDI Limited

Geristore Syringeable Dual-Cure Resin-Ionomer
DenMat Holdings, LLC

Conventional Glass Ionomer Restorative Material

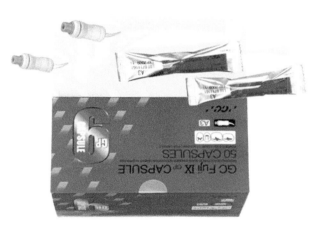

GC Fuji IX GP Capsule glass ionomer
GC America Inc.

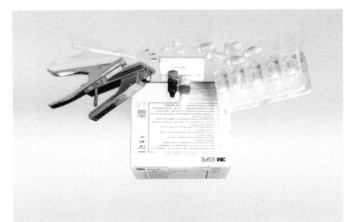

Ketac Silver Aplicap glass ionomer restorative
3M ESPE Dental Products

Compomers

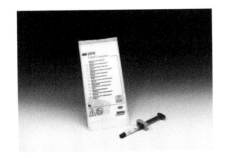

F2000 Compomer restorative
3M ESPE Dental Products

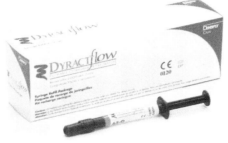

Dyractflow Flowable Compomer
Restorative
DENTSPLY Caulk

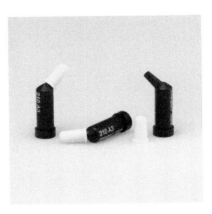

Compoglass F advance performance
compomer restorative
Ivoclar Vivadent Inc.

Customized Provisionals

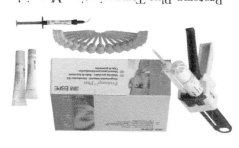

Protemp Plus Temporization Material
3M ESPE Dental Products

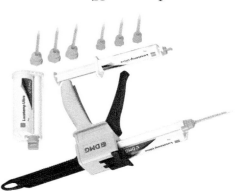

Luxatemp Ultra
DMG America

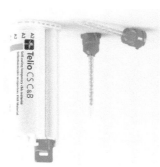

Telio CS C&B temporary
crown and bridge material
Ivoclar Vivadent Inc.

Heat-Activated Dental Acrylic Resins

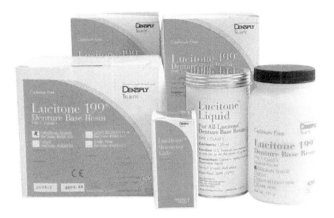

Lucitone 199 Denture Base Resin
DENTSPLY International Inc.

Chemically-Activated Dental Acrylic Resins

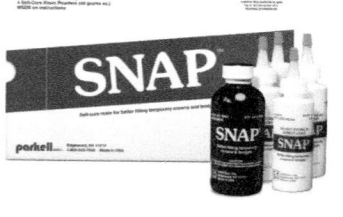

SNAP temporary bridge and
crown material
Parkell Inc.

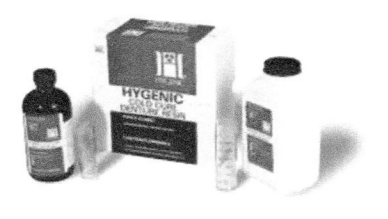

Hygenic Cold Cure Denture
Resin
Coltène/Whaledent Inc.

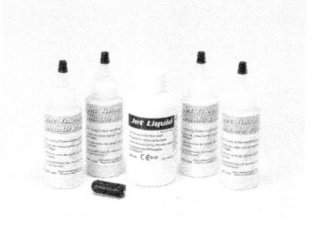

Jet Tooth Shade Powder
self-curing acrylic resin
Lang Dental Manufacturing
Company, Inc.

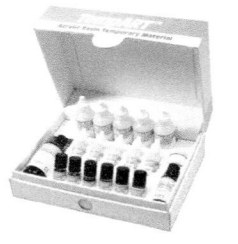

TempART Acrylic
Resin
Sultan Healthcare

Light-Activated Dental Acrylic Resins

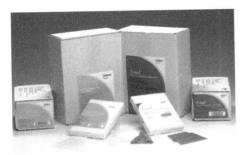

Traid TruTray VLC Custom Impression
Tray Material
DENTSPLY International Inc.

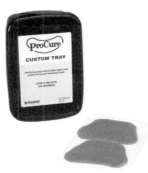

ProCure Custom Tray
material
Keystone Industries

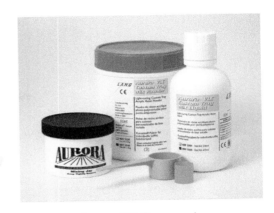

Aurora VLC tray resin
Lang Dental Manufacturing Company, Inc.

Intermediate Restorative Material (IRM)

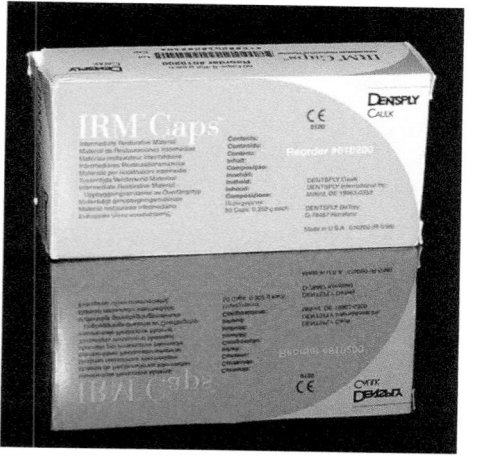

IRM Caps Intermediate Restorative Material
DENTSPLY Caulk

Block-Out Resin

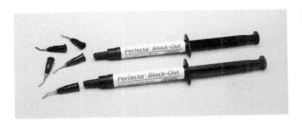

Perfecta Block-Out resin
Premier Dental Products

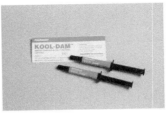

KOOL-DAM kit
PULPDENT Corporation

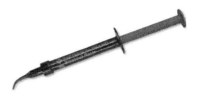

Patterson Brand Blockout Resin
Patterson Dental Supply

Hydrogen Peroxide

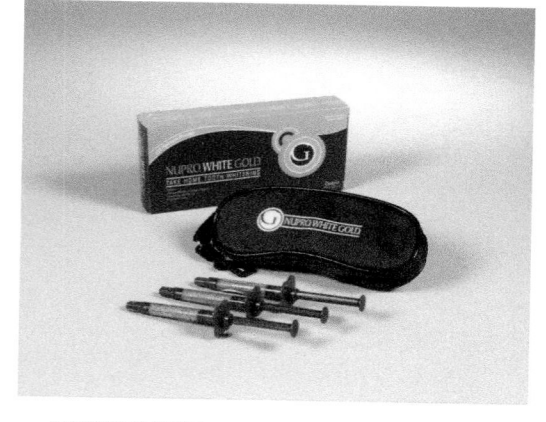

NUPRO White Gold Take Home Tooth
Whitening system
DENTSPLY Professional

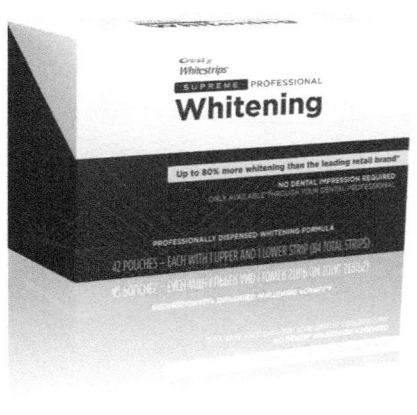

Crest Whitestrips Supreme
Professional Whitening
Proctor & Gamble Company

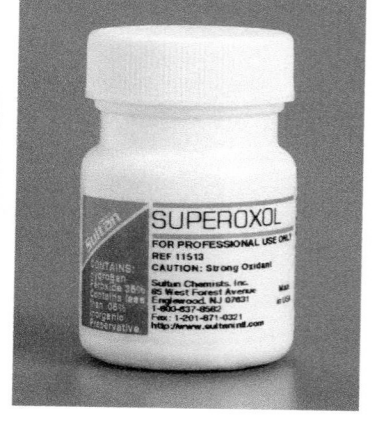

Superoxol in-office teeth
whitening
Sultan Healthcare

Carbamide Peroxide

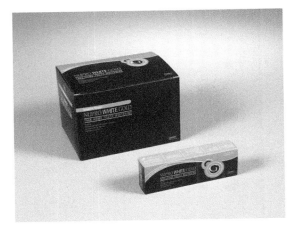

NUPRO White Gold Take Home Tooth Whitening system
DENTSPLY Professional

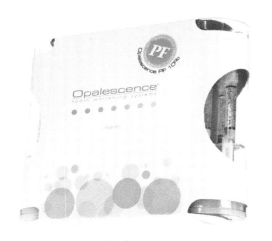

Opalescence
Ultradent Products, Inc.

Sodium Perborate

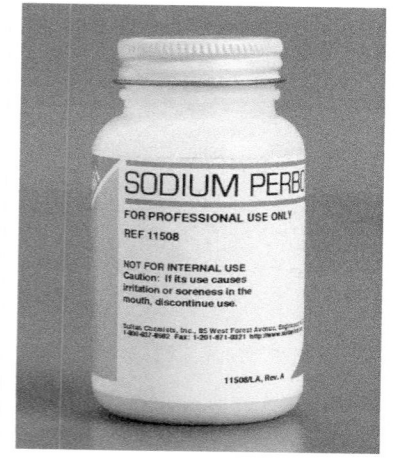

Sodium Perborate teeth whitening
Sultan Healthcare

In-Office Professionally Applied Whitening

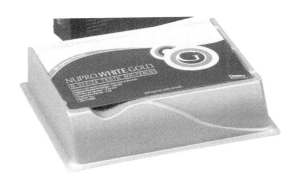

NUPRO White Gold Tooth Whitening System
DENTSPLY Professional

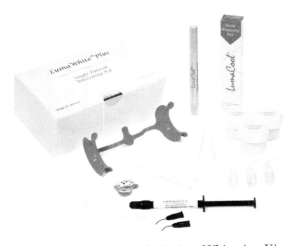

LumaWhite Plus Single Patient Whitening Kit
LumaLite, Inc.

Zinc Oxide Eugenol Cement "Temp Bond"

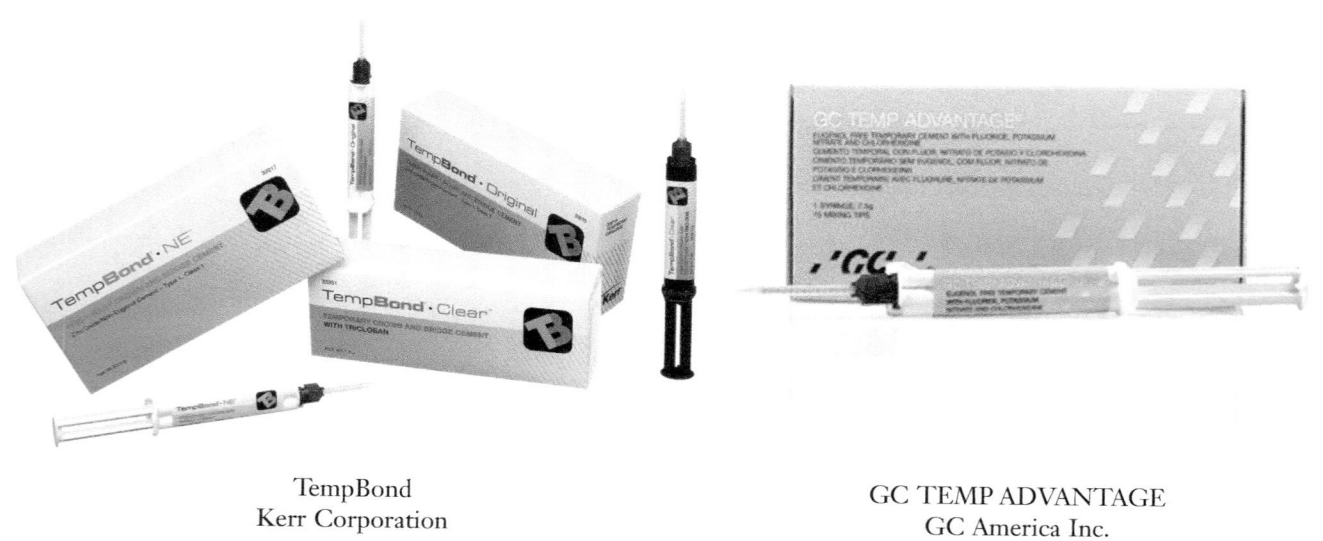

TempBond
Kerr Corporation

GC TEMP ADVANTAGE
GC America Inc.

Zinc Phosphate Cement

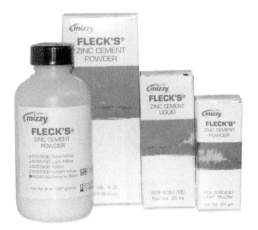

Fleck's Zinc Cement
Mizzy Inc.

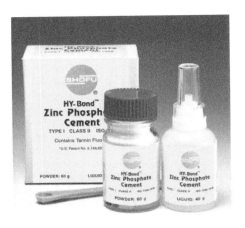

HY-Bond Zinc Phosphate Cement
Shofu Dental Corporation

Zinc Polycarboxylate Cement

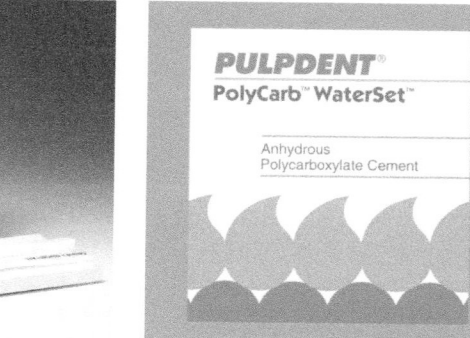

HY-Bond Polycarboxylate
Cement
Shofu Dental Corporation

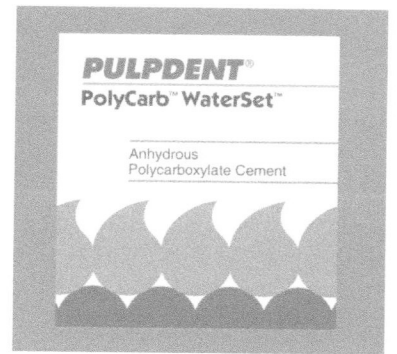

PolyCarb WaterSet
PULPDENT Corporation

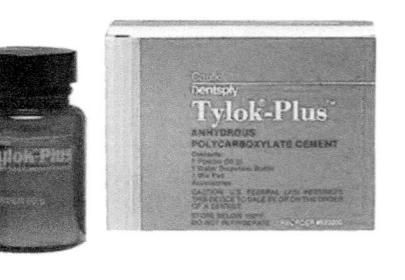

Tylok-Plus
DENTSPLY Caulk

Glass Ionomer Cement

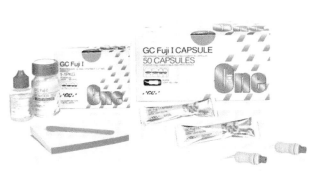

GC Fuji I glass ionomer luting cement
GC America Inc.

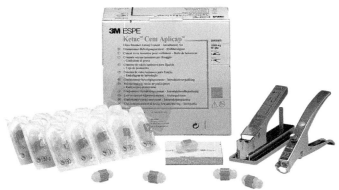

Ketac Cem Aplicap Glass Ionomer Luting Cement
3M ESPE Dental Products

Resin Modified Glass Ionomer Cement

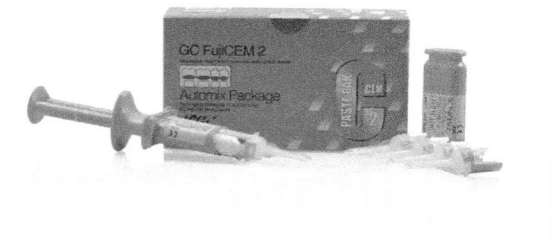

GC FujiCEM 2
GC America Inc.

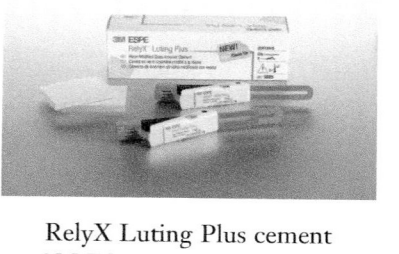

RelyX Luting Plus cement
3M ESPE Dental Products

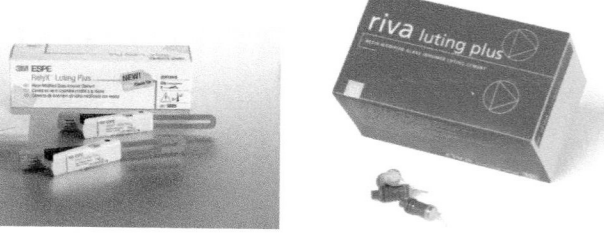

Riva Luting Plus cement
SDI Limited

Resin Cement

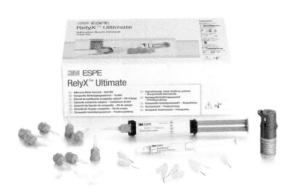

RelyX Ultimate Adhesive Resin Cement
3M ESPE Dental Products

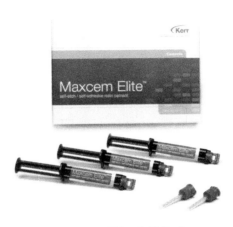

Maxcem Elite Self-Etch
Kerr Corporation

Polyether

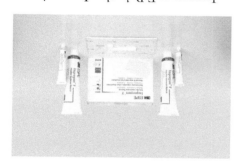

Impregum F Polyether Impression
Material
3M ESPE Dental Products

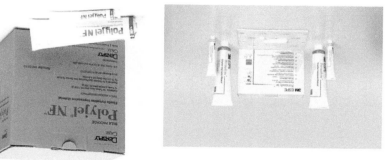

Permadyne Polyether Impression
Material
3M ESPE Dental Products

Polyjel NF Elastic Polyether
Impression Material
DENTSPLY Caulk

Addition Silicone "Vinyl Polysiloxane"

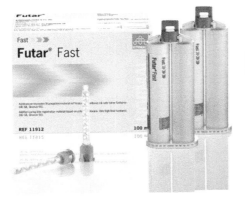

Futar Fast bite registration material
Kettenbach GmbH & Co.

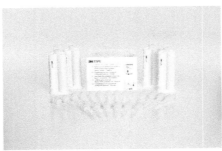

Imprint II Garant Quick Step
3M ESPE Dental Products

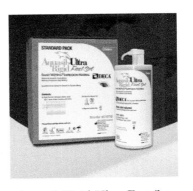

Aquasil Rigid Ultra Fast Set
Smart Wetting Impression
Material
DENTSPLY Caulk

Addition Silicone "Putty Vinyl Polysiloxane"

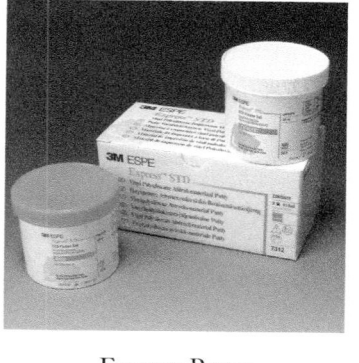

Express Putty
3M ESPE Dental Products

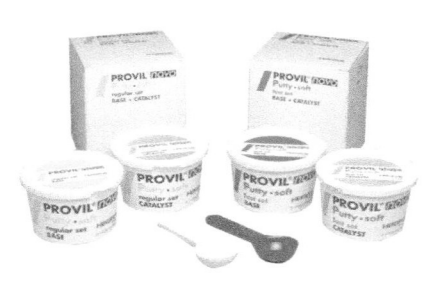

PROVIL Novo Putty Soft VPS
impression material
Heraeus Kulzer, LLC

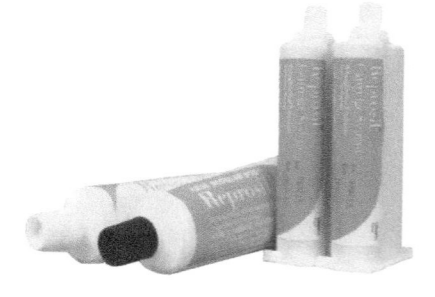

Reprosil Hydrophilic Vinyl Polysiloxane
Impression Material
DENTSPLY Caulk

Polysulfide

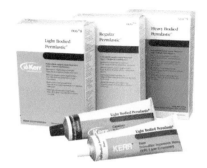

Permlastic
Kerr Corporation

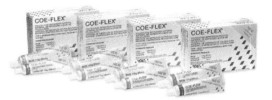

COE-FLEX Polysulfide Impression Material
GC America Inc.

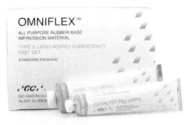

OMNIFLEX All Purpose Rubber
Base Impression Material
GC America Inc.

Impression Plaster

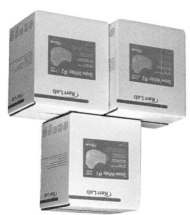

Snow White model plaster
KerrLab Corporation

Impression Compound

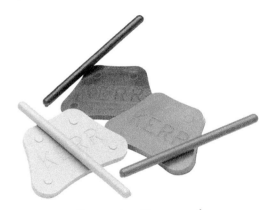

Impression Compound
Kerr Corporation

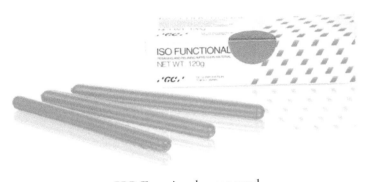

ISO Functional compound
GC America Inc.

Zinc Oxide Eugenol Impression Material

Bosworth Plastopaste Zinc Oxide
Eugenol Impression Paste
Harry J. Bosworth Company

COE-FLO
GC America Inc.

ZONE edentulous impression paste
Cadco Dental Products, Inc.

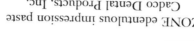

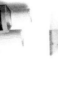

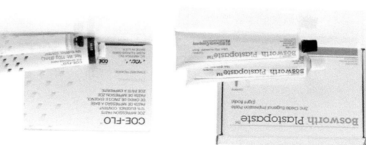

Alginate

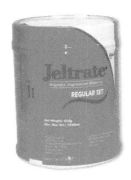

Jeltrate Alginate Impression
Material
DENTSPLY Caulk

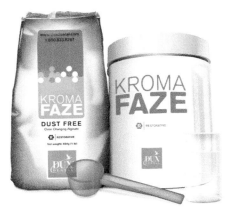

KromaFaze alginate impression
material
DUX Dental

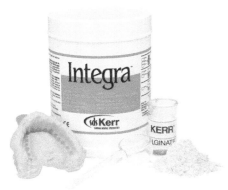

Integra alginate
Kerr Corporation

Model Plaster

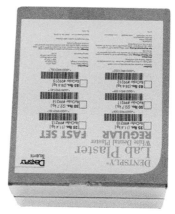

Lab Plaster
DENTSPLY International
Inc.

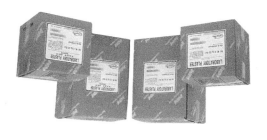

Laboratory Plaster
Whip Mix Corporation

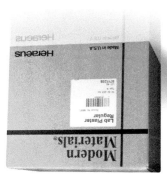

Modern Materials Lab Plaster
Heraeus Kulzer, LLC

Dental Stone

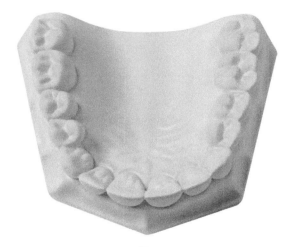

Buffstone
Whip Mix Corporation

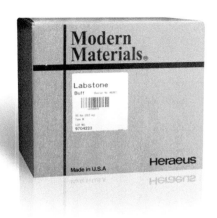

Modern Materials Labstone gypsum
Heraeus Kulzer, LLC

High-Strength Improved Stone

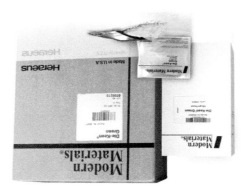

Modern Materials Die-Keen Green
Heraeus Kulzer, LLC

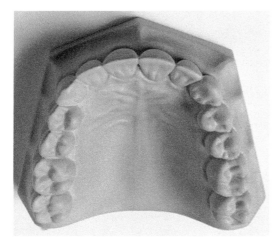

Prima-Rock High Strength Die Stone
Whip Mix Corporation

Inlay Wax

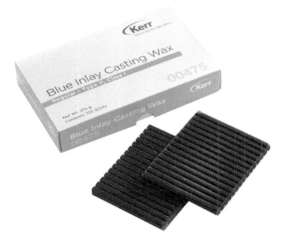

Blue Inlay Casting Wax
Kerr Corporation

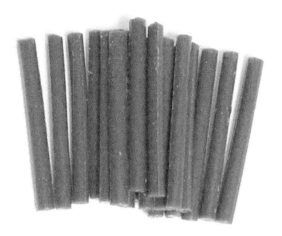

Maves Inlay Wax Sticks
Maves Co., Inc.

Casting Wax

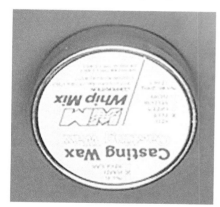

Regular Casting Wax
Whip Mix Corporation

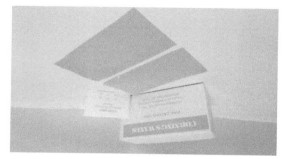

Corning's Waxes Pink Casting Wax
Corning Waxes Co., Inc.

Baseplate Wax

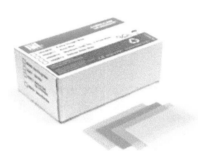

Baseplate Wax
Coltène/Whaledent Inc.

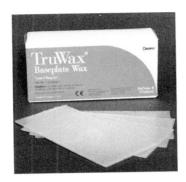

TruWax Baseplate Wax
DENTSPLY International
Inc.

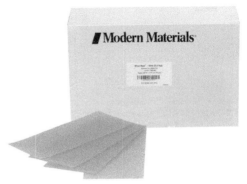

Modern Materials Shur Wax
Heraeus Kulzer, LLC

Boxing Wax

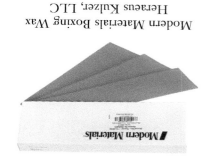

Modern Materials Boxing Wax
Heraeus Kulzer, LLC

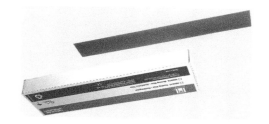

Boxing Wax
Coltène/Whaledent Inc.

Utility Wax

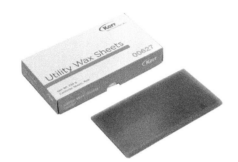

Utility Wax Sheets
Kerr Corporation

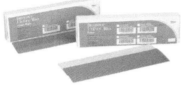

Utility Wax
DENTSPLY International Inc.

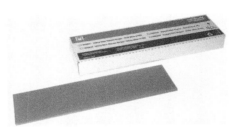

Utility Wax
Coltène/Whaledent Inc.

Sticky Wax

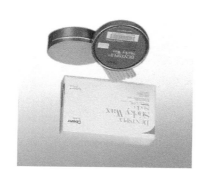

DENTSPLY Sticky Wax
DENTSPLY International Inc.

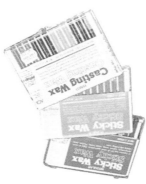

Regular Sticky Wax
Whip Mix Corporation

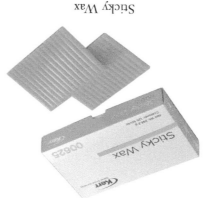

Sticky Wax
Kerr Corporation

Bite Registration Wax

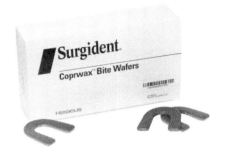

Surgident Coprwax Bite Wafers
Heraeus Kulzer, LLC

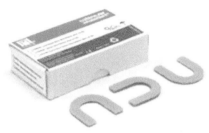

Bite Wafers
Coltène/Whaledent Inc.

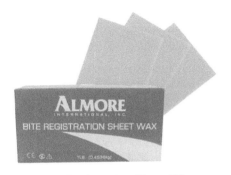

Bite Registration Sheet Wax
Almore International, Inc.

Aluminum Oxide

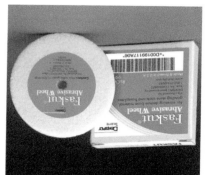

Faskut Abrasive Wheel aluminum oxide lathe wheel
DENTSPLY International, Inc.

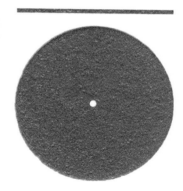

Elite Aluminum Oxide Discs
Dedeco International, Inc.

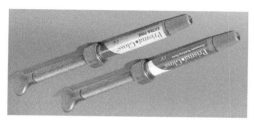

Prisma Gloss
DENTSPLY Caulk

Silicon Carbide

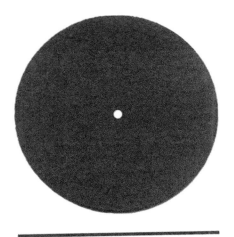

Elite Silicon Carbide Discs
Dedeco International, Inc.

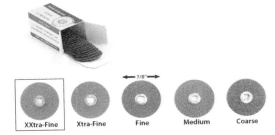

Moore's Discs paper brass center abrasive
discs—silicon carbide
E.C. Moore Company, Inc.

Pumice

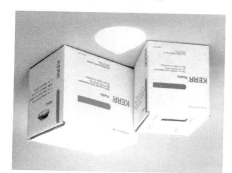

Pumice powder
Kerr Corporation

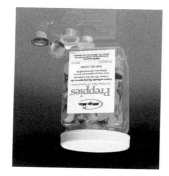

Preppies Unit Dose Flour of Pumice
Paste
Whip Mix Corporation

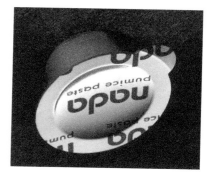

Nada pumice paste—fluoride free
Preventive Technologies, Inc.

Rouge

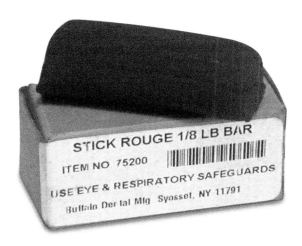

Red rouge stick
Buffalo Dental Manufacturing Company

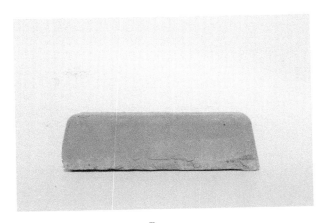

Rouge
California Dental Products

Cuttle

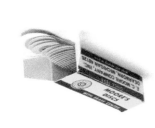

Fine

Medium

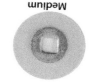

Coarse

Moore's Discs paper brass center abrasive discs—cuttle
E.C. Moore Company, Inc.

Garnet

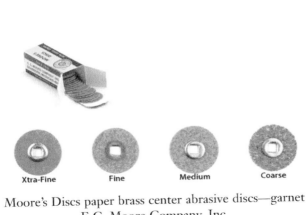

Moore's Discs paper brass center abrasive discs—garnet
E.C. Moore Company, Inc.

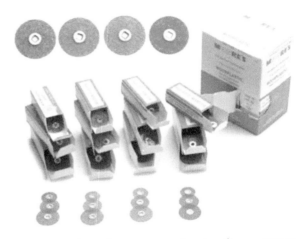

Moore's plastic brass center abrasive discs—garnet
E.C. Moore Company, Inc.

Emery

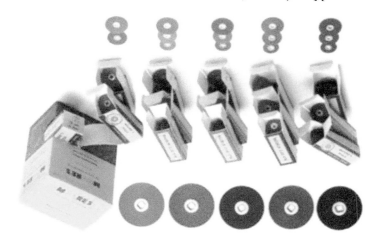

Moore's paper brass center abrasive discs—emery
E.C. Moore Company, Inc.

Silex

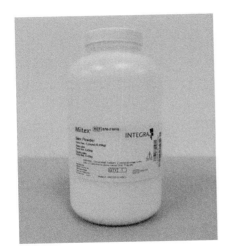

Miltex Silex Powder
Integra Miltex

Tin Oxide

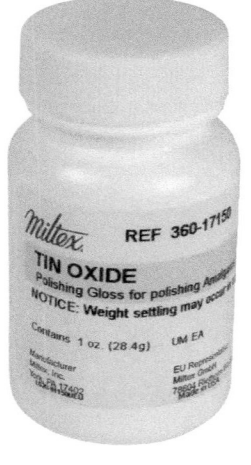

Tin Oxide
Integra Miltex

Prophylaxis Paste

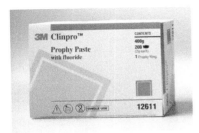

Clinpro Prophy Paste with fluoride
3M ESPE Dental Products

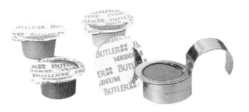

Butler prophy paste
Sunstar Americas, Inc.

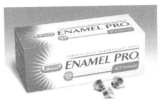

Enamel Pro professional prophylaxis paste
Premier Dental Products

Digital Impression Powder

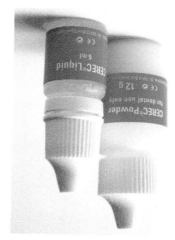

CEREC Powder for optical impressions
Vident

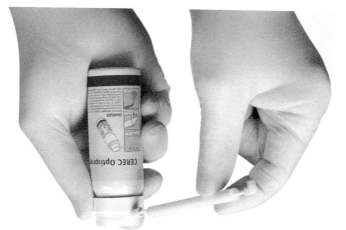

CEREC Optispray
Sirona Dental Systems, LLC

Acidulated Topical Fluoride

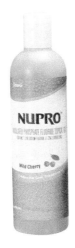

NUPRO Acidulated Phosphate Fluoride Topical Gel
DENTSPLY Professional

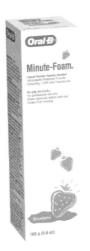

Oral-B Minute-Foam Topical Fluoride Foaming Solution
Proctor & Gamble Company

Neutral Topical Fluoride

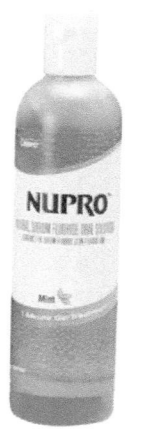

NUPRO Neutral Sodium Fluoride (NaF) Oral Solution
DENTSPLY Professional

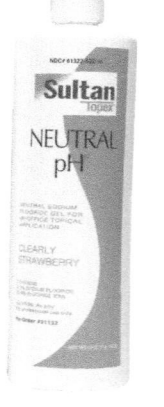

Topex Neutral pH Topical Gel
Sultan Healthcare

Fluoride Varnish

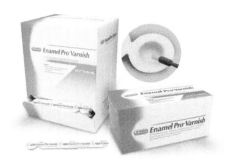

Enamel Pro Varnish 5% Sodium Fluoride
Varnish
Premier Dental Products

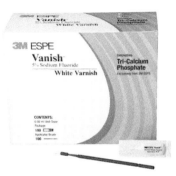

Vanish 5% Sodium Fluoride
White Varnish with
Tri-Calcium Phosphate
3M ESPE Dental Products

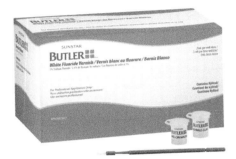

Butler White Fluoride Varnish
Sunstar Americas, Inc.

Sealants

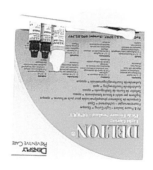

DENTSPLY
DELTON Light Curing
Pit & Fissure Sealant
Professional

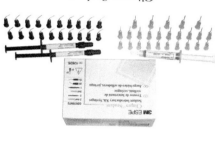

Clinpro Sealant
3M ESPE Dental Products

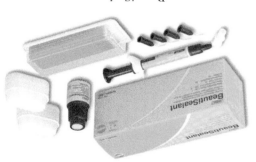

BeautiSealant
Shofu Dental Corporation

Gutta Percha

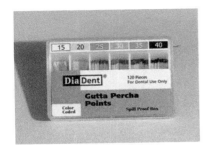

Gutta Percha Points
DiaDent Manufacturing Inc.

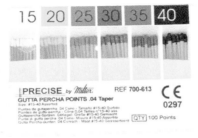

Precise Gutta Percha Points
Integra Miltex

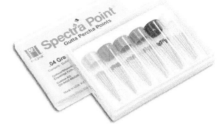

Hygenic SpectraPoint Gutta Percha
Points
Coltène/Whaledent Inc.

Root Canal Sealer

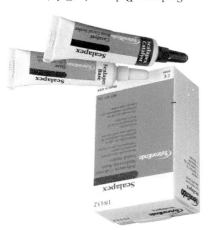

Sealapex Polymeric Calcium
Hydroxide Root Canal Sealer
Sybron Dental Specialties Inc.

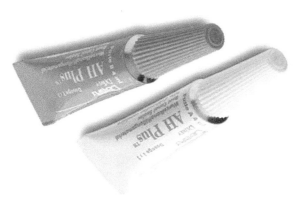

AH Plus root canal sealer
DENTSPLY Maillefer

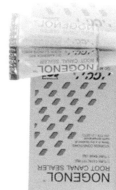

Nogenol Root Canal
Sealer
GC America Inc.

Root Canal Lubricant

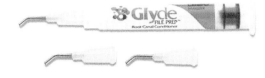

Glyde File Prep Root Canal Conditioner
DENTPLY Maillefer

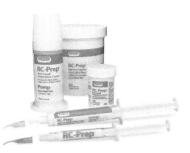

RC-Prep Root Canal Preparation
Cream
Premier Dental Products

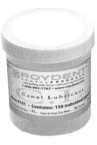
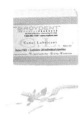

C.L. Canal Lubricant
Roydent Dental Products

Periodontal Dressing

Barricaid
DENTSPLY Caulk

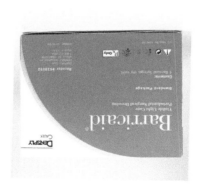

PerioCare periodontal dressing
Pulpdent Corporation of America

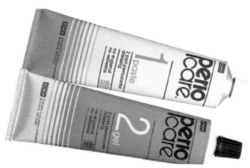

Coe-Pak Automix NDS
Periodontal Dressing material
GC America Inc.

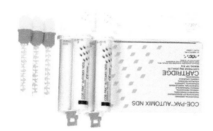

Alveolar Dressing

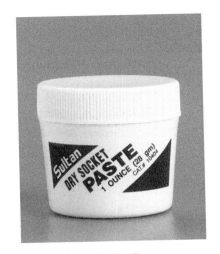

Dry Socket Paste
Sultan Healthcare

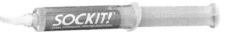

SockIt Dressing
MCMP

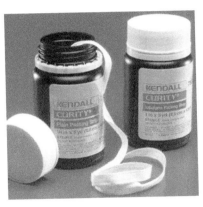

Curity Iodoform Packing Strips
Kendall

Index

Note: Page numbers followed by *f* indicate figures.